Eden's Health Plan –

Go Natural!

Live Long Enough to Fulfull Your Destiny

by

Mark and Patti Virkler

What people are saying about Eden's Health Plan – Go Natural!

"At last a helpful, complete and balanced look on natural health and healing which doesn't ignore or avoid the spiritual side of the equation. Written from a warm Christian perspective with sensitive wisdom without the preachy flavor." Dr. Albert Zehr

"I went down four dress sizes!" K.F.

"I found your book, *Eden's Health Plan – Go Natural!* to be packed full of valuable suggestions for better health. Great statements such as 'Cancer is not a disease. It is a symptom of an insufficient immune system' are of inestimable value, emotionally, physically and even financially. I am glad to recommend it." Rev. Herman Riffel

"An excellent book! I pray it will be widely received." Maurice Fuller

"Finally, a book about holistic health from a Christian perspective. This is a valuable resource book for those who want to improve their health, but don't know where to begin. I will recommend it to all who are seeking to know God's will for healthy living." Valerie C. Wilson R.M.T. (Registered Massage Therapist)

"It's wonderful to have had the opportunity to read your book (*Eden's Health Plan – Go Natural!*). Looks to be a very comprehensive and excellent program. I read it with great fascination and believe that it is going to be an excellent blessing to the Body of Christ." Dr. Stan E. DeKoven, President Vision Christian College

"Most people who write books on health address the body, a few go a step further and incorporate the mental and emotional components to health, and Mark and Patti have gone even further...they have added the spiritual dimension. That is unique in the health field — this book is unique! We are spirit, soul, and body — a triune being — true health needs God's truth in all areas. I highly recommend this book to you, because Mark and Patti have grasped all three!" Gale Chapple, Lay Counselor and Facilitator; Entrepreneur

Eden's Health Plan –

Go Natural!

Live Long Enough to Fulfull Your Destiny

by

Mark and Patti Virkler

God's covenant of health:

And he cried unto the LORD; and the LORD showed him a tree, which when he had cast into the waters, the waters were made sweet: there He made for them a statute and an ordinance, and there He proved them, And said, If thou wilt;

1. diligently hearken to the voice of the LORD thy God, and

2. wilt do that which is right in His sight, and

3. wilt give ear to His commandments, and

4. keep all His statutes,

   I will put none of these diseases upon thee, which I have brought upon the Egyptians: for I am the LORD that healeth thee (literally, Lord your health).

   —Exodus 15:25,26

In this book we will try to learn how to live in this wonderful covenant of health which God has made with His people!

Destiny Image Publishers, Inc.®
P.O. Box 310
Shippensburg, PA 17257
1-800-722-6774

"Speaking to the Purposes of God for this Generation
and for the Generations to Come"

ISBN 1-56043-138-5

First Printing: 1994   Second Printing: 1995

For Worldwide Distribution
Printed in the U.S.A.

> **IMPORTANT NOTICE:**
> The information and procedures contained in this book are not intended as a substitute for consulting your physician. Any attempt to diagnose and treat an illness should come under the direction of a physician who is familiar with nutritional therapy.

Foreword

In this volume, Mark Virkler has compiled a wealth of effective health information. The value of this book goes far beyond a writer's intellect to reflect on scriptural teaching that is put to the test in the real world. His work reflects the wisdom of having lived out the restoration of God's Health Plan for our lives.

The words of this book are effective tools for positive change in our lives. The ideas of this book work best when they are applied through the leading of the Holy Spirit, for the Spirit will guide us into all truth.

I recall the story of a primitive man who stumbled across a pair of prescription eyeglasses. As he was closely examining the glasses, he happened to look through them. Immediately he noticed that his vision had greatly improved. This realization led him to believe that he had found the answer to all the world's eyesight problems. But as you would imagine, only a small number of the people he tried the eyeglasses on were actually helped.

We need to remember the experience of this primitive man when seeking God's wisdom for our health. This book contains much sound and safe information, but its personal application, as in all issues of your life, should be led and confirmed by the Holy Spirit.

By applying scriptural truths to diet and lifestyle management, Mark shows how to prevent or deal with many of the common health problems of this age. But he also goes beyond this to reveal how we should glorify God in our bodies by living healthy and vital lives.

Mark has done the body of Christ a great service in compiling this information. I am convinced through my many years of practice that this book holds valuable treasures we need to apprehend the fullness of health that God has for us all.

Frank J. King, N.D., D.C.

Acknowledgements

We would like to express our gratitude to the following people:

To Claire Hudson and Diane Hale, for the hours they put into proofreading the manuscript;

To Linda Basta, Laura Besch, Keith Carroll, Gale Chapple, Maurice Fuller, Roger Miller, Herman Riffel, and Gary Tatar for their careful reading of the manuscript and helpful suggestions.

To Kimberly Bright Cassano, Dr. Frank King, Albert Ocker, Valerie Wilson, and Dr. Albert Zehr for their expertise and encouragement.

Dedication

This book is dedicated with love to our children, Charity and Joshua. May the Spirit of purity rule in every area of your lives, giving you physical, emotional and spiritual wholeness. May you live long enough in vibrant health to fulfill the awesome destinies God has in mind for you. We love you!

Table of Contents

Introduction

Questions concerning health

Wouldn't it be nice if God's children were the healthiest people in the world? Wouldn't it be nice if they were the most vivacious, active, spontaneous and creative? Wouldn't it be nice if they lived the longest, accomplished the most and became the most outstanding leaders the world has ever seen? Wouldn't it be nice if they didn't get the diseases common to the rest of the world because they knew how to live sanctified lives according to the Word of God? I wonder if that was God's plan? I wonder if such a thing is possible? What do you think?

The current dismal scene

My heart wept as I walked through the airport, passing the lethargic, shuffling crowd with a listless gait. Some were standing in line waiting to purchase "food" which they fully intended to put in their mouths, poisoning their entire systems and making them even more lethargic. Many probably do not know that the United States Surgeon General has said that half of the people who die in America every year die because of what they eat. I have a good idea what their destiny holds. They will likely find themselves with degenerative diseases requiring several stays in the hospital, during which they will experience humiliating, invasive and mutilating surgery, followed by an early and pain-filled death. All of this could be avoided, if only they knew.

They are led as sheep to the slaughter — lambs without a shepherd, or at least without a good shepherd — innocently assuming that if the food is available for purchase, it must be safe to eat. They do not know that the law of the land requires that processed food be dead before it is sold. Most of the "living" food is sold at the perimeter of the store.

They innocently assume that the doctor and the Food and Drug Administration (FDA) are looking after their health. And some doctors are, because they are seekers after truth. They are courageous men and women who stand against the tide of our times and offer wholeness of body and soul. However, many simply adopt the outdated and ineffective remedies of the past, and the pronouncements of the FDA, trusting its honesty and accuracy. They do not know that greed and a limited world-view corrupt such agencies. So they are led as sheep to the slaughter, lambs without a shepherd.

How I wish I could tell them what I have learned about health and nutrition! I wish they could taste how full of health and vitality I have become since I began to practice the simple principles delineated in this book. I wish I could convince them to turn from the path they have so trustingly chosen. How I wish I could spare their lives from the tragedy which is before them, and indeed which many of them **are already walking in**. As I travel the country, I find that "everyone" is sick! This ought not to be in a nation as prosperous as ours! How I wish I could place in everyone's hands a copy of this book and say, "Try everything it suggests for thirty days. See how you feel after **only one month**." I know they would be rejuvenated. I believe their health would be renewed. I am convinced that many inoperable and degenerative diseases would be reversed, and in some cases, would go into complete remission by following the simple, non-invasive, inexpensive solutions presented in this book.

However, I can't convince them to change. That is the work of the Holy Spirit. I can't undo the effects of wrong training in just a few minutes. Many are not even asking me for that kind of help. Only about 20 percent of people are seekers after truth. Another 40 percent will embrace truth when it is presented to them and there is a great enough need in their lives. The rest will not embrace truth, even though they are in critical need and it is right there before them.

I can offer the truths I have seen to you, the reader. You are taking the time to read, to look and to listen. I pray you have an open heart. I pray you have the heart of a learner. I pray you are a **seeker of truth**. And more than that, I pray that your life is **submitted** to Truth, so that when it (that is, He, Jesus) confronts you, you have chosen to yield your life to His claims upon you. For indeed the Good Shepherd, the Shepherd of our souls, has said that He is truth and that His truth "shall set you free" — if you will heed it! How tragic it is for one to know the truth and not act upon it. How tragic it is to walk through life without even discovering the way of life. My prayer is that neither of these tragedies would happen to you, dear reader.

Life is too short. It is too precious to squander in listlessness, lethargy, sickness and disease. It was not intended to be lived this way. It was intended to be lived in divine health, filled with joy and ecstasy, vitality and abundance. It was designed to be fulfilling beyond measure. And mine has become so. After losing these wonderful, precious gifts for several years, they have been restored by discovering and practicing the truths that are recorded on the pages that follow.

And so I offer you an abundance of health, life, energy and vitality by following a few simple, biblically grounded rules of health care. Try them for thirty days, and I believe you will never return to your old ways of living. Wouldn't it be worth a thirty-day test, just to see? Can we live 80, 100, even 120 years in vital health? I think we can. Why not read and decide for yourself?

Chapter 1

An Unhealed Nation!

My early, unwise decision

I remember thanking God for giving me a strong, vibrant physical body which was hardly ever sick. I remember thinking at age twenty that, when I got older and my body began breaking down, I would study health and healing and gain a better understanding of how to maintain the wonderful gift of health with which God had blessed me. That may not have been one of my smarter decisions because once you damage a gift as precious as your health, it can be very difficult to restore it to its original strength. You see, the most common cause of death in the United States is heart disease. Every year, 1.2 million people have a heart attack. Fifty percent of them die. Fifty percent of those who die never knew they were sick. They may have gone for a medical check-up and received a clean bill of health. The first sign of heart problems for many is death. Heart disease is a socially acceptable way to die. And it leaves millions of widows and orphans every year.

Twenty years later

Well, by the time I was forty, my body had broken down. I was full of stress, had become fat, and my energy level was always low. Even after eating a huge meal, I still felt low energy and continued to eat and eat. But it didn't seem to help. My high energy was gone. I felt gaseous pain in my upper stomach after every meal. I was beginning to feel some chest pains which made me wonder about the condition of my heart. My vitality was gone. My resistance to disease had waned and I was easily susceptible to germs and sicknesses. Stress would throw my neck and back out of place regularly. My toe would get inflamed with infection. My intestines had picked up parasites from travel abroad, and I was an all-around mess.

I discerned it was time to begin studying health and healing, but by now I had lost my energy to do so! By 5:00 in the afternoon, I only had enough energy to sit on the sofa, eat M&M's and watch television, trying not to move too much because my system was exhausted from the day's work. And I was the person who had always worked full steam until 11:00 at night!

So I went to my doctor, and had a complete physical. He said I was in great shape except that my cholesterol was a bit high. I went back a year later and he again said I was fine except that my cholesterol was even higher (274) and that my triglycerides were about 300. That, he informed me, put me at maximum risk for coronary disease, and he recommended I go on a strict diet right away.

Discovering motivation and strength to change

That got my attention a fair bit. Having a wonderful, loving wife and two dynamic teen-agers, I did not think it would be too smart to die, leaving them to fend for themselves. So I discovered the motivation I needed to get moving and begin taking care of myself physically. At the same time, I was picking up additional energy and motivation through some herbs and chromium I had begun taking. They were not only giving me energy, but also weight loss, muscle gain, suppression of appetite and suppression of desire for sweets. They increased the blood flow to my brain, so I felt more alert, and helped in the digestion of food.

I regained enough energy and motivation to begin a one-year study on diet, disease and divine healing. I read more than seventy books, experimented with their suggestions on my own body, went on a seven-day fast, lost twenty-seven pounds, sixty-three points of cholesterol and seven inches around my waist. I felt my energy and vitality and physical frame restored to that of twenty years earlier when I was only twenty years of age, and I am still improving every day, even at the writing of this book.

So I decided to share with you what I have learned so far. I am sure it is incomplete knowledge, but it is considerably more than I have ever had before. And I am convinced it is enough to help many others who may also be struggling with health problems. I am not a doctor of medicine by training, so my findings must be tempered by that fact.

Those familiar with my writing are aware that I never present a problem without also presenting a solution. My practical German nature sees problems as challenges to be overcome, and I am only satisfied when I have analyzed a situation, discovered solutions that work in my life, and clearly communicated my findings to others so their lives can be enhanced as well. Therefore, this book will contain references to specific products and disciplines which I have found effective in dealing with specific needs. This doesn't mean that these products are the only ones available which can do these things. It just means that they are the ones I have chosen to use. You are certainly encouraged to do your own research and find alternatives that meet the same criteria, if you'd like. The information I am presenting is my testimony, offered to assist those who face similar problems but who don't have the time, resources, or inclination to do intensive research.

Another motivation to study health

I have been frustrated for years by the fact that I, and others in the body of Christ who believe in prayer for divine healing, see only limited results to our prayers. Sometimes prayer works miraculously well. Sometimes it appears to work for a while, and sometimes it doesn't seem to work at all. Even Kathryn Kuhlman said that she did not understand why some were healed and others were not. Well, I certainly didn't either, and I found it incredibly frustrating.

I believe that healing is an incredibly complex issue, that there are many reasons why a person can become sick, and many avenues which can be used to make one healthier. It is often a matter of matching the right solution to the discerned need. That takes a bit of knowledge and discernment and anointing — more than I had. Well, my year's study in the area of health has given me many more answers than I have ever had before, and I am convinced I can help many more people than I have before when it comes to the area of physical health. I don't for a minute believe I have learned it all. I am a learner along the road of life, and look forward to learning much in the years to come in this area, as well as others.

A researcher

I discovered that a recent investigation by a Senate subcommittee revealed that the average physician in the United States receives less than three hours of training in nutrition during four years of medical school, and that less than three percent of the licensing exam questions are concerned with nutrition.[1] I was astounded by the realization that the year of research I had just completed may have given me greater knowledge than the average doctor has on the relationship of diet to disease. I somehow assumed that doctors would focus heavily on the fuel our bodies take in, since our bodies are complex, intricate engines burning this fuel at a constant temperature of 98.6 degrees and **designed to repair themselves IF GIVEN THE PROPER TOOLS!** Obviously, if we are taking in the wrong fuel, our engines will sputter and could malfunction, and our bodies' ability to repair themselves will be impaired.

Detours taken by Western medicine

1. Focus on cure rather than prevention.

Western medicine has focused much more on cure of disease than on prevention. Rather than trying to keep me healthy, doctors are trained to help maintain me when I become sick. And they will not maintain me primarily through diet or natural means, but through synthetic pharmaceutical medicines which often have severe side effects. Students in medical school study pathology (i.e. sickness) rather than health.

2. Corruption of major medical establishments.

Pharmaceutical companies have become big business and, when linked with the FDA, are able to maintain an almost complete stranglehold on any and all **natural means** of physical rejuvenation. Instead, they fill the market with high-cost synthetic drugs and procedures which in may leave the patient in worse shape than before receiving the treatment. The corruption which I found documented in my research shocked and sickened me. It was a major factor in my decision to **take charge of my own health,** which has been one of the best decisions I have ever made.

Benjamin Rush, M.D. and signer of the Declaration of Independence, foresaw years ago what has happened to us when he wrote, "Unless we put medical freedom into the Constitution, the time will come when medicine will organize into an undercover dictatorship ...the Constitution of this Republic should make special provision for medical...as well as religious freedom."[2]

I am not against doctors. I object to the abuse of power by doctors who try to limit individuals' freedom to choose the methodology of healing which they believe is best for themselves.

3. Over-emphasizing one theory of disease over all others.

Another over-emphasis in Western medicine is the result of the pendulum-swing from one theory of disease to another. Until the late 1800's, doctors did not wash their hands before examining patients. It was common practice for medical students to go straight from their work in the morgue to hospital wards to examine their living patients. Of course, the diseases which had killed those in the morgue were spread to the patients. Hospitals became breeding grounds for disease. Ignaz Semmelweis (1818-1865) discovered that the simple ritual of washing one's hands between patients had tremendous benefit. Yet, when he tried to convince the medical community of the mass murder it was perpetrating on innocent victims entrusted to its care, he was laughed at, ridiculed to scorn, and fired from his position in the hospital (even though his hand-washing procedure reduced mortality rate in his ward to about 1%). After his firing, his hand-washing procedures were dropped and mortality rates again soared. He instituted his procedures in other hospitals with the same results — a drastic reduction in the spread of disease, and ridicule and rejection. It was not until after his death that medical science accepted his procedures.[3]

Now, of course, medical science has accepted the "germ theory of disease." However, it has done so to the almost total exclusion of the truth that if we provide our bodies with a healthy immune system, **our bodies' defense artillery** can fight off most diseases successfully themselves. Now, medical experts laugh in derision at anyone who would suggest that proper food, vitamins and nutrition can build a powerful immune system which could in itself destroy cancer. It is scary to see the arrogance and intolerance mankind has of any and all opposing views. Lord, deliver us from our pride and arrogance so we can be seekers of truth, even if that means our own views and our financial security may be threatened.

No wonder God put medical care in the hands of the priests (Lev. 14). I am sure it was with the hope that, as spiritual leaders, they would demonstrate humility, righteousness, and a godly honoring of truth, regardless of what it cost them. Perhaps this needs to happen once again. Perhaps the individuals in church leadership themselves need to become spiritual enough to be willing to **lose their lives**, and pet doctrines, and job security, for the truth. They must be willing to be open-minded **searchers** after truth. If church leaders won't meet these criteria (and often they won't), how can we ever expect others to? The church sets the standard for the world in which we live.

But hasn't Western medicine increased our lifespan?

From 1870 to 1970 the average lifespan in the United States increased substantially. However, this was primarily because infant mortality declined from 150 to about 10 deaths per 1000. Once a person safely reaches age 45 (i.e. past the somewhat dangerous child-bearing years for women), the actual increase of lifespan is only six years in the last century.[4] Not exactly spectacular, considering all the research and money that has gone into medicine, and the awesome hospitals in every community, and the billions of dollars spent annually on health care.

Cancer

I also learned that I was not the only one sick in America. We are a nation of sick people. Even after spending hundreds of billions of dollars on cancer research and treatment, the percentage of people in America who get cancer each year continues to grow. Now, about one in three will be afflicted with this terrifying disease — an exciting statistic, since I have four in my family and some of my grandparents died of cancer, so cancer "runs in the family". If you are a woman, your chance of getting cancer in 1900 was 1 in 40. By 1990 it had become 1 in 2.6 (for women).[5] That is a 1500% increase for women in just 90 years. I find it amazing that we cannot get a handle on cancer when some cultures of the world have practically no cancer. Why can't we simply observe their diet and lifestyle, and experiment with it to see if it would reduce cancer in our culture?

Some doctors have done this and have written about their findings. Among them is Dr. Max Gerson who wrote **A Cancer Therapy — Results of Fifty Cases** and **The Cure of Advanced Cancer by Diet Therapy**, a summary of thirty years of clinical experimentation. In 1946 he testified before a United States Congressional subcommittee on his success in curing advanced cancer through diet. Gerson died in 1959 and was eulogized by Nobel Prize winner Albert Schweitzer (Gerson had cured his wife of lung tuberculosis after all conventional treatments had failed): "I see in him one of the most eminent geniuses in the history of medicine." What a pity that Gerson's simple, inexpensive way of treating cancer through diet has not yet caught on. We could have saved billions of dollars, and untold suffering and agony, and needless bodily mutilation in so many millions of lives. Gerson's clinic for the nutritional healing of cancer still functions (The Gerson Institute) and his books, tapes, newsletters and diet plan are still available (619-472-7450). The Gerson Institute has tremendous expertise and success in dissolving cancerous tumors through diet therapy. If I had cancer, I would surely go on the diet Dr. Gerson teaches in his books and stay on it until I was healed.

What absolutely amazed me is that the diet Gerson recommends, as well as that recommended by other doctors who heal the body of various diseases through diet, is the same diet that God gave man in Genesis 1:29. A shocking revelation struck me, that —

the Genesis diet heals!!!

"And God said, Behold, I have given you every herb bearing seed, which is upon the face of all the earth, and every tree, in the which is the fruit of a tree yielding seed; to you it shall be for meat" (Genesis 1:29).

In a later chapter we will explore what foods are contained in this diet and why they are so healing. In the rest of this chapter, I will briefly show how modern scientific studies have proven over and over again that the Genesis diet which is low in fat, low in cholesterol and high in fiber, is the healthiest diet in the world.

Many great historical figures have adopted this diet. They include Daniel, Albert Einstein, Ralph Waldo Emerson, St. Francis, Benjamin Franklin, John Milton, Isaac Newton, Plato, Albert Schweitzer, Socrates, Henry David Thoreau, Voltaire, H.G. Wells, and John Wesley, to name just a few.

Osteoporosis

Americans are sick with more than continuously rising cancer rates. An epidemic fifteen to twenty million persons in the United States are affected by osteoporosis, costing $4 billion annually for diagnosis and care of these suffering people. About 1.3 million fractures attributed to osteoporosis occur annually in people forty-five years and older. Approximately 100,000 wrist fractures occur each year from osteoporosis. One hundred ninety thousand hip fractures occur annually at a cost of more than one billion dollars. Eighty percent are in postmenopausal women. At least 15,000 women die each year as a direct result of hip fractures. Of those who recover, only 25 percent regain full mobility. The diagnosis and care of people suffering from this disease has become a four billion dollar-a-year health business in the United States.[6]

This entire tragedy, with all its accompanying pain and suffering, is preventable by consuming the Genesis diet. We will show how and why in a later chapter.

Atherosclerosis

Atherosclerosis can be thought of as sores on the many miles of arteries in your body, which are caused by slivers of cholesterol which injure the inside of the linings. Build-up occurs within the arteries until we have a stroke or heart attack. Then we know our arteries are rotten.

As soon as you change your diet, more cholesterol flows out of your arteries than flows in, and its accompanying diseases immediately go into regression. You experience the reversal of atherosclerosis. Within hours of changing your diet, you reduce your risk of dying of heart disease. I changed my diet, removing three-quarters of the meats and dairy products and two-thirds of the sugar, and within 90 days my cholesterol had dropped 65 points. (I was also taking Shackley's Heart Plan Formula, Cholestrex capsules from a health food store, and eating Fiber One cereal from the grocery store.)

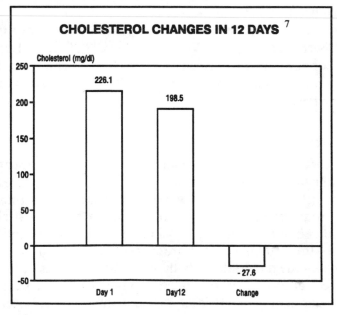

CHOLESTEROL CHANGES IN 12 DAYS [7]

Cholesterol (mg/dl)

226.1

198.5

- 27.6

Day 1   Day12   Change

Cholesterol is not cement. It can be reduced through lowering fat intake. On the Genesis diet, which John McDougall recommends in **The McDougall Program**, his patients average a nearly 28 point drop in cholesterol in twelve days!

Atherosclerosis is epidemic in America. Studies show that at least one out of three major coronary arteries is narrowed by 50 percent or more in approximately half of the high-risk men below age forty.[8,9] Autopsies of 300 men killed in the Korean conflict (average age of 22 years) showed that 77 percent of them had atherosclerotic disease in the arteries that supplied the heart muscle, known as the coronary arteries. Eight had almost complete or complete blockage of at least one of the essential arteries that had kept their hearts beating long enough to allow them to be killed in action.[10]

The good news is that **the day** one begins the Genesis diet, his arteries begin to cleanse and heal themselves.

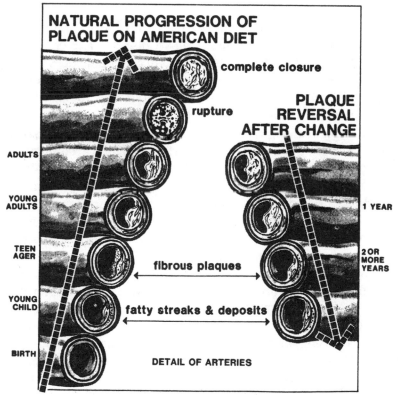

NATURAL PROGRESSION OF PLAQUE ON AMERICAN DIET

complete closure

rupture

PLAQUE REVERSAL AFTER CHANGE

ADULTS

YOUNG ADULTS

1 YEAR

TEEN AGER

fibrous plaques

2 OR MORE YEARS

YOUNG CHILD

fatty streaks & deposits

BIRTH

DETAIL OF ARTERIES

11

Cholesterol

Just as a grade on a test does not really tell what you know but it is an indicator, so cholesterol does not tell you the state of your health, but it, too, is a good indicator. It is one of the most reliable indicators we have of the overall state of our health. The average cholesterol in America is between 210 and 220. You don't want to be average because the average male in America has a greater than 50 percent chance of dying from heart disease. A decrease in your cholesterol of about 60 points will decrease your risk of dying of heart disease about five fold. (I just reduced mine 65 points, from 274 to 209, in 90 days!) Many studies have proven that when your cholesterol gets below 150, you are essentially immune to heart disease. In Framington, MA more than 4000 people were followed for 40 years and it was found that when cholesterol was 150 or less, the people did not get heart disease.

Heart Disease

Cholesterol levels in one's bloodstream are probably the strongest indicator of one's risk of developing heart disease. The chart on the following page shows that as one's cholesterol goes up, so does incidence of heart disease. The second chart shows that in only three weeks on a cholesterol-free diet, one can drop cholesterol about 100 points.

It was almost unbelievable to me how much better I felt when my cholesterol dropped 65 points. It was hard to believe that a change in lifestyle could do so much in such a short time. When accumulation of cholesterol is great, as it was for me, the large deposits of cholesterol throughout the body are released into the blood and in that way keep the level elevated for a long time. Eventually, after several years of eating proper foods, the cholesterol deposits may be depleted and the cholesterol levels will begin to fall again. At 150 or 160 there is essentially no chance of developing heart disease. That is my personal goal. I did have my cholesterol checked about three months after my initial cholesterol drop, and even though I had been on a low-cholesterol/low-fat and high-fiber diet, my cholesterol level had not dropped any more. It had even gone up a few points. I was very encouraged to learn that an inner cleansing of my artery walls was occurring, although my cholesterol may not fall any further the next two years. However, I will be cleaning up the damage I have been doing to my body for the last forty years. That understanding is comforting. Plus, every day I seem to have more energy. I suspect that as the arteries are being cleansed

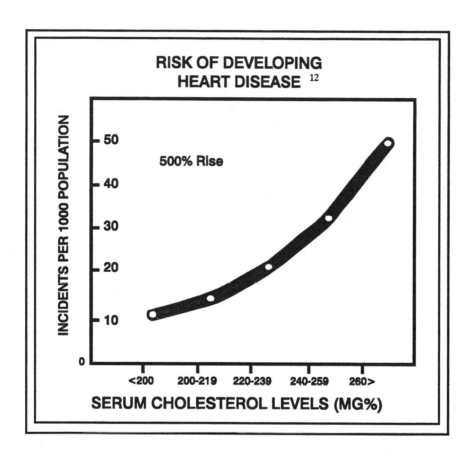

RISK OF DEVELOPING
HEART DISEASE [12]

500% Rise

INCIDENTS PER 1000 POPULATION

SERUM CHOLESTEROL LEVELS (MG%)

of their plaque build-up, more blood is flowing, carrying more oxygen to every part of my body, and thus a sense of being "more alive" continues to permeate every part of my being day by day. Do you think I'm thrilled and excited? Try it, you'll love it!

Bypass surgery is a $5 billion a year business that earns many surgeons $1 million and more annually. Each year 200,000 trusting patients are sent to these surgeons, asking to have their clogged arteries bypassed.[14] Major complications of one kind or another affect about 13 percent of the patients.[15] Studies show that nearly 100 percent of the patients who are placed on the heart-lung machine suffer some form of brain injury.[16-18] Almost every review of the results of by-pass surgery has concluded that this surgery does not save lives when compared with simply giving patients drugs that relieve their angina.[19-23] A five year review of the survival rates of those receiving bypasses showed 82 percent still alive, while 80 percent of those who were simply treated with medicines were still alive.[24]

One-quarter of by-pass patients return to the hospital within six months of their operation. Nearly 60 percent of the readmissions are for chest pains and other heart-related complaints.[25] Evidence from researchers from the Cardiovascular Laboratories, Harvard School of Public Health, has shown that even with severe coronary artery disease, good medical care along with changes in diet and lifestyle will give equal or better results than surgery.[26] As a matter of fact, the primary reason people submit to by-pass surgery is to alleviate chest pain. Open heart surgery does relieve that pain. However, a low-fat diet is also highly effective and much less harmful, not to mention less expensive. In patients using such a dietary treatment, chest pain episodes are decreased by 91 percent in only twenty-four days without the

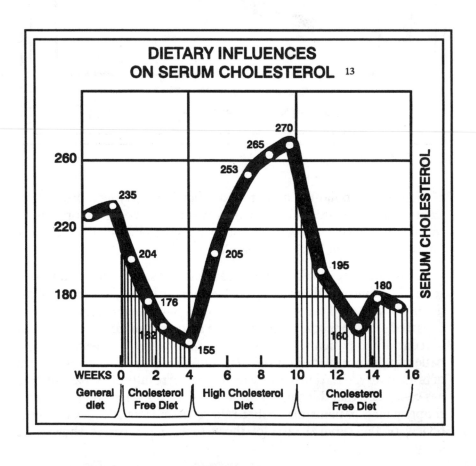

$25,000 - $37,000 price tag and painful foot-long incision across the victim's chest.[27] Doesn't this sound more reasonable? I think I prefer simply sticking to the Genesis diet.

Hypertension

About 23 million American adults have high blood pressure. They make about 25 million visits to their doctors per year, and drugs are prescribed in 89 percent of those cases.[28] People with high blood pressure have twice the chance of dying from anything at all, twice the chance of closure of the arteries in the legs, three times the chance of dying from heart attacks, four times the chance of heart failure, seven times the chance of having a stroke.[29-31]

It is not a coincidence that the societies where blood pressure remains the same throughout adult life are the same as those where blood levels of cholesterol, triglycerides, and uric acid are also low, and obesity is uncommon. All these positive characteristics are common to people who follow the Genesis diet, or a diet based on grains, potatoes, and other starchy foods. Normal blood pressure in these countries is 110/70. That is what I have chosen to aim for.

Diabetes

One in twenty people in the United States has diabetes.[32] Childhood-onset diabetes represents less than five percent of the cases of diabetes. The rest are adult-onset. Diabetics have earlier and more severe complications from atherosclerosis, which lead to kidney failure, heart attacks and strokes.[33-36] The typical high-fat, low-carbohydrate, and low-fiber American diet is a primary culprit in adult onset diabetes. The Genesis diet, which is low-fat, high-carbohydrate and high in fiber, is a primary healer of adult onset diabetes.

Arthritis

Arthritis is a term that refers to signs and symptoms of inflammation in any joint in the body. Osteoarthritis is the most common of all types of arthritis. At least 85 percent of persons aged 70 to 79 have diagnosable osteoarthritis, which compromises the quality of life they can live. An estimated 180,000 people in the United States are bed or wheelchair invalids because of this common disease.[37] Osteoarthritis and osteoporosis, another bone disease common in the United States, are rare among people in underdeveloped countries where they are much more likely to be eating the Genesis diet than are Americans.[38]

Investigators at Wayne State University Medical School fed a fat-free diet to six patients suffering from rheumatoid arthritis. They found complete remission of the disease in all six patients within seven weeks. The symptoms recurred within seventy-two hours when either vegetable oil or animal fats were introduced into their diets. Chicken, beef, cheese, coconut oil, and safflower oil all caused severe arthritis in these patients. The investigators concluded that "dietary fats in the amounts normally eaten in the American diet cause inflammatory joint changes seen in rheumatoid arthritis."[39] Again, the Genesis diet heals and the American diet wounds.

Urinary Disease

Various urinary diseases can also be avoided or healed through the Genesis diet. For example, in the United States, vegetarians (people who eat the Genesis diet), have about half the incidence of kidney stones as the general population.[40]

Kidneys are damaged by excessive protein consumption, a high fat diet and excessive intake of Vitamin C (more than 12,000 mg/day). Twenty years ago, the World Health Organization determined that a 176 pound adult needed only 1 1/3 ounces, or 40 grams of protein daily. (That was actually 30% higher than their studies indicated. The extra was added as a safety factor). Since the body cannot store excess protein, any extra that is consumed must be excreted, putting tremendous overload on one's kidneys. The average American consumes 90 to 150 grams of protein daily (or three or four times more than the body needs or can use).

In 1984, Drs. William E. Mitch and MacKenzie Walter published in the New England Journal of Medicine a study of 24 patients who had chronic kidney failure. They were treated with a low-protein diet containing only 20 to 30 grams of mixed quality protein, plus some specialized low-acid protein supplements. Seventeen of the patients had slower progression of their kidney failure, and seven of these patients had no progression or even reversal of their kidney failure.

Prostate Problems

The prostate is a gland which only men have and is associated with the sex act. Prostate enlargement and subsequent urinary problems occur for the majority of men over age 40, including urgent and frequent need to urinate, slow stream, hesitance and pain in urination.

This enlargement is caused most largely by the American high fat diet. In Thailand, Japan, Taiwan and Ceylon, where the average dietary fat consumption falls between 25 and 45 grams per day, the average death rate from prostate cancer is two or less deaths per 100,000 men. But in the United States, New Zealand, Australia and most of the countries in Western Europe, where the average fat consumption is between 120 and 160 grams per day, the death rate from prostate cancer is 12 to 18 per 100,000 men. Fully 165,000 new cases of prostate cancer are diagnosed every year in the U.S. and 35,000 men die of it.[41]

Between 1984 and 1990, the incidence of prostate operations increased sixteen fold. Currently, 400,000 operations at $12,000 each are being done annually in the U.S.[42] According to Dr. John Wennberg of the Dartmouth Medical School, the death rate is as high as 1.3% (one death per 77 procedures), 8 percent of the men having the procedure have complications requiring hospitalization within three months, and 5 percent of them develop impotence. Also, 20 percent of all men need to repeat the procedure within eight years. Other reports show that, for 15 percent of the patients, symptoms can return in about a year and 4 percent of the patients suffer from incontinence.[43]

The Swedes generally do not treat prostate cancer. Their five year survival rate was 92 percent. The survival rate of those who have radical surgery is 90 percent.[44]

Certain herbs such as saw palmetto and its extract Serenoa have been shown to relieve prostate problems, increasing urine flow rate by 38% as compared to only a 16% increase with Proscar.[45] Proscar is the more expensive drug ($75 per month) approved by the FDA to treat prostrate problems. Plus the following warning comes with the drug Proscar: "Exposure of Women — Risk to Male Fetus — It is not known whether the amount of finasteride that could potentially be absorbed by a pregnant woman through either direct contact with crushed Proscar tablets or from the semen of a patient taking Proscar can adversely affect a developing male fetus....Therefore, because of the potential risk to a male fetus, a woman who is pregnant or who may become pregnant should not handle crushed Proscar tablets; in addition, when the patient's sexual partner is or may become pregnant, the patient should either avoid exposure of his partner to semen or he should discontinue Proscar."[46]

I think I will go on a low fat diet instead, and if necessary take the natural herb saw palmetto and some zinc. All men should purchase and read Prostate Report by Dr. Julian Whitaker (1-800-777-5005). From the same number you may also order various natural non-toxic non-surgically-invasive remedies for prostate problems.

And If You Have to Go to the Hospital...

Make sure to take your own low-fat, high-fiber diet with you because the typical hospital menu is laden with fat and cholesterol, and with fiber-deficient foods. These foods will keep you sick longer and often contribute to the development of new diseases.

Summary

After carefully notating thousands of scientific studies in his three volumes, The McDougall Plan, McDougall's Medicine, and The McDougall Program, John McDougall, M.D. presents us with a list of the diseases which are caused by a "rich" western diet, and which can be healed by the Genesis diet. His list follows.

Eating Ourselves into Early Graves by Way of Painful, Debilitating Diseases

I believe the issue of whether the American diet heals or destroys has been settled in the same way the issue on smoking was settled: by a Surgeon General's report. The Surgeon General of the United States said in 1988 that **over one million deaths in the United States are caused by what we eat**. So out of the two million people who die in the U.S. each year, half of them **take their own lives, in slow suicide** through what they eat day after day. Unbelievable! The Surgeon General said that five of the ten leading killer diseases in the United States are caused by what we eat. These include heart disease, cancer, stroke, atherosclerosis and diabetes.[48]

In December of 1990, Dr. Sullivan, the Secretary of Health and Human Services, reported a rise of 11 percent in the cost of providing health care to the nation. It is generally estimated that the health care costs of the United States will reach a staggering figure of $1.6 trillion by the year 2000 and will consume 28 percent of our Gross National Product by the year 2010. Of course, there is no solution in sight.

DISEASES CAUSED BY
A "RICH" WESTERN DIET

Systemic Diseases	Bowel Disorders	Cancers
Allergies	Appendicitis	Breast
Arthritis	Colitis	Colon
Atherosclerosis	Constipation	Kidney
Diabetes (Adult)	Diarrhea	Pancreas
Gout	Diverticulosis	Prostate
Heart Attacks	Gallstones (cholesterol)	Testicle
Hormone Imbalances	Gastritis	Uterus (body)
Hypertension	Hemorrhoids	
Kidney Failure	Hiatus Hernia	
Kidney Stones	Indigestion	
Multiple Sclerosis	Malabsorption	
Obesity	Polyps	
Osteoporosis	Ulcers	
Strokes		

* Diet is a primary causative factor in all the above diseases and it is *controllable*. (Heredity is also a primary factor, but it is not under our control.) Smoking, alcohol, lack of exercise, and "stress" are secondary factors which are also controllable. A primary factor must be present for a disease to develop; a secondary factor aggravates the disease process after the development has begun.

* *Diet and lifestyle changes are the most effective treatment for chronic forms of the diseases listed in the first tow columns,* far surpassing in results any drug or surgical therapy according to scientific and medical literature. This should not surprise you; what causes disease promotes disease. If you eliminate the cause, then the body's healing mechanisms can take over, resulting in improvement or recovery. The effect of diet on cancers is yet to be determined.[47]

Health Through Prevention

Perhaps it is time we take care of people with a new set of principles which are simple, cost-effective, medically-proven and sensible. May I suggest the following: the Genesis diet, exercise, nutritional and herbal supplements as necessary, clean air, pure water, adequate sunshine, attitudes of faith, hope and love, occasional fasting, and prayer for healing when necessary. I believe that by practicing these we can probably live to 100 years of age in excellent health and great spirits. Perhaps that would give us enough years to develop the talents and anointings necessary to become mighty world changers for Jesus. We can become those who participate in discipling nations. We shall pursue these possibilities in future chapters.

A Preview of Where This Book Will Take You

Everything we will study about in this book heals by doing at least one of three things: 1) it detoxifies the body; 2) it builds the immune system; or 3) it nourishes the cells. We must become constantly aware of how the things we do promote either overall health or sickness by either honoring or dishonoring the above principles. **The bottom line** is that degenerative diseases (and the aging process itself) can be slowed, halted, and even reversed by doing simple things: 1) detoxifying your body, 2) strengthening your immune system and 3) nourishing your cells.

This is true because the growth of mutated cells within one's body causes degenerative diseases (cancer, etc.) and the aging process. A strong lymphatic system (immune system) eats up and destroys mutated cells before they can multiply into growths, diseases and aging symptoms. Well-nourished cells will stay strong and healthy and perform their assigned jobs without breaking down. This book will reference many scientific studies along with testimonies which show that:

We can detoxify the body by
* Eating the Genesis diet
* Breathing pure air
* Drinking pure water
* Eating vital food
* Excreting waste from the intestines quickly
* Using herbs wisely

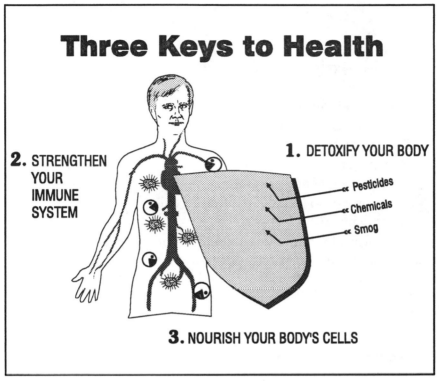

Three Keys to Health

2. STRENGTHEN YOUR IMMUNE SYSTEM

1. DETOXIFY YOUR BODY

« Pesticides
« Chemicals
« Smog

3. NOURISH YOUR BODY'S CELLS

* Super-foods
* Removing toxic chemicals from surfaces which one touches
* Taking vitamins and minerals
* Taking antioxidants
* Fasting
* Praying for healing.

We can strengthen our immune systems by
* Eating the Genesis diet
* Praying for healing
* Begin healed of past emotional traumas
* Living in a spirit of faith, hope and love
* Exercising
* Eating vital food
* Taking vitamins and minerals
* Using herbs wisely
* Taking aloe vera

* Taking Pycnogenol
* DHEA
* Superfoods
* Co-enzyme Q10.

We can nourish our cells by

* Eating the Genesis diet
* Eating superfoods
* Breathing pure air
* Taking vitamins and minerals
* Drinking 7 or 8 glasses of pure water daily
* Co-enzyme Q10.

We will expand each of these points in future chapters, bringing you to an excellent understanding of how our bodies fight cancer and disease, and how we can make sure that our immune systems win, over and over again! A healthy immune system that is not swamped with toxins **can** fight off diseases successfully! Awesome!

For Further Reading

The following books about diet and disease provided much of the research behind this chapter and are an ESSENTIAL PART of everyone's education. THESE BOOKS CAN SAVE YOUR LIFE. All are by John A. McDougall M.D. and Mary A. McDougall.

The McDougall Plan

Over 1/4 million copies sold. 330 pages of unbelievable insight into what the Genesis diet is and why it works so well, and comparison of various cultures around the world which do and do not follow this diet. 108 recipes. Nearly 1000 scientific studies are notated which give overwhelming evidence that the Genesis diet heals.

McDougall's Medicine: A Challenging Second Opinion

Here are the reasons why present therapies are not improving or prolonging life for most people. Nearly a thousand scientific studies are notated which give overwhelming evidence that the Genesis diet reduces cancer, osteoporosis, atherosclerosis, heart disease, hypertension, diabetes, arthritis and kidney disease.

Required Reading for All Men

The Prostate Report: Prevention and Healing by Julian Whitaker M.D.

This book will give you in clear, simple language an understanding of prostate problems and easy, natural things you can do to prevent and heal them. Order book and three bottles of product for $39 from 1-800-777-5005 (Phillips Publishing, Inc.).

Concerning Institutional Corruption

The Healing of Cancer: The Cures — Cover-ups — and the Solution Now! by Barry Lynes.

This book documents the corruption of the Food and Drug Administration (FDA), the National Cancer Institute (NCI), the American Medical Association (AMA), and the American Cancer Society (ACS). It will shock you and **convince you to take responsibility for your own health care,** which is a good lesson for each of us to learn. One quote from the book by Herbert L. Ley, Jr., M.D., **former Commissioner of the FDA,** is as follows: "People think the FDA is protecting them — it isn't. What the FDA is doing and what people think it's doing are as different as night and day."[49]

Concerning Current Cancer Therapies

Options: The Alternative Cancer Therapy Book by Richard Walters

This book overviews 23 alternative approaches to treating cancer and provides resource addresses for these therapies.

References

[1] John A. McDougall and Mary A. McDougall, *The McDougall Plan* (Clinton, NJ: New Win Publishing, Inc., 1983), p. 7.

[2] Swope, Mary Ruth, *Green Leaves of Barley* (Melbourne, FL: National Preventive Health Services, 1987), p. 22.

[3] Rosen, George, "Semmelweis, Ignaz Philipp," *The World Book Encyclopedia*, 1989 ed.

[4] McDougall, *The McDougall Plan*, p. 182.

[5] Hosking, Richard, *You and Super Blue Green Algae*, (cassette) Klamath Falls, OR: Cell Tech, 1993.

[6] John A. McDougall, *McDougall's Medicine: A Challenging Second Opinion* (Clinton, NJ: New Win Publishing, Inc., 1985), p. 62.

[7] John A. McDougall, *The McDougall Program* (New York: Penguin Books, 1990), p. 29.

[8] Welch C. Cinecoronary Arteriography in Young Men. Circulation 42:647, 1970, as cited by John A. McDougall, *McDougall's Medicine: A Challenging Second Opinion*, p. 99.

[9] Page I. Prediction of coronary heart disease based on clinical suspicion, age, total cholesterol and triglycerides. Circulation 42:625, 1970, as cited by McDougall, *McDougall's Medicine: A Challenging Second Opinion*, p. 99.

[10] Enos W. Pathogenesis of coronary disease in American soldiers killed in Korea. JAMA 158:912, 1955, as cited by McDougall, *McDougall's Medicine: A Challenging Second Opinion*, p. 99.

[11] McDougall, *McDougall's Medicine: A Challenging Second Opinion*, p. 100.

[12] McDougall, *The McDougall Plan*, p. 66.

[13] McDougall, p. 67.

[14] Preston T. Marketing an Operation. Atlantic December 1984 p. 32, as cited by McDougall, *McDougall's Medicine: A Challenging Second Opinion*, p. 145.

[15] Kuan P. Coronary artery bypass surgery morbidity. J Am Coll
Cariol 3:1391, 1984, as cited by McDougall, *McDougall's Medicine:
A Challenging Second Opinion*, p. 146.

[16] Henriksen L. Evidence suggestive of diffuse brain damage
following cardiac operations. Lancet 1:816, 1984, as cited by
McDougall, *McDougall's Medicine*, p. 147.

[17] Aberg T. Release of adenylate kinase into cerebrospinal fluid
during open-heart surgery and its relation to postoperative
intellectual function. Lancet 1:1161, 1982, as cited by McDougall,
McDougall's Medicine, p. 147.

[18] Henriksen L. Brain hyperfusion during cardiac operations:
Cerebral blood flow measured in man by intra-arterial injection of
xenon 133: Evidence suggestive of intraoperative microembolism.
J Thorac Cardiovasc Surg 86:202, 1983, as cited by McDougall,
McDougall's Medicine, p. 147.

[19] Braunwald E. Editorial retrospective. Effects of coronary-artery
bypass grafting on survival; implications of the randomized
Coronary-Artery Surgery Study. New England Journal of
Medicine 309:1181, 1983, as cited by McDougall, *McDougall's
Medicine*, p. 147.

[20] McIntosh H. The first decade of aortocoronary bypass grafting,
1967-1977: a review, Circulation 57:405, 1978, as cited by
McDougall, *McDougall's Medicine*, p. 147.

[21] Hampton J. Coronary artery bypass grafting for the reduction of
mortality: an analysis of the trials. Br Med J 289:1166, 1984, as
cited by McDougall, *McDougall's Medicine*, p. 147.

[22] Grondin C. Late results of coronary artery grafting: is there a flag
on the field? J Thorac Cardiovasc Surg 87:161, 1984, as cited by
McDougall, *McDougall's Medicine*, p. 147.

[23] Kolata G. Consensus on bypass surgery: in most cases, the
operation has not been shown to save lives, but patients do say
they feel better after surgery. Science 211:42, 1981, as cited by
McDougall, *McDougall's Medicine*, p. 147.

[24] The Veterans Administration Coronary Artery Bypass Surgery
Cooperative Study Group. Eleven-year survival in the Veterans
Administration randomized trial of coronary bypass surgery for

stable angina. N Engl J Med 311:1333, 1984, as cited by McDougall, *McDougall's Medicine*, p. 148.

[25] Stanton B. Hospital readmissions among survivors six months after myocardial revascularization. JAMA 253:3568, 1985, as cited by McDougall, *McDougall's Medicine*, p. 150.

[26] Podrid P. Prognosis of medically treated patients with coronary-artery disease with profound ST-segment depression during exercise testing. N Engl J Med 305:1111, 1981, as cited by McDougall, *McDougall's Medicine*, p. 151.

[27] Ornish, D. Effects of stress management training and dietary changes in treating ischemic heart disease. JAMA 249:54, 1983, as cited by McDougall, *McDougall's Medicine*, p. 158.

[28] Cypress B. Medical therapy in office visits for hypertension: National Ambulatory Medical Care Survey. 1980. National Center for Health Statistics Advanced Data, No. 80, July 22, 1982, as cited by McDougall, *McDougall's Medicine*, p. 171.

[29] Kannel W. Should all mild hypertension be treated? Yes. In: Lasagna L. (ed) *Controversies in Therapeutics* Lasagna L (eds.) Philadelphia: W. B. Saunders Co, 1980. p-299, as cited by McDougall, *McDougall's Medicine*, p. 172.

[30] Fry J. Deaths and complications from hypertension. *J Roy Coll Gen Pract* 25:489, 1975, as cited by McDougall, *McDougall's Medicine*, p. 172.

[31] Evans P. Relation of longstanding blood-pressure levels to atherosclerosis. Lancet 1:516, 1965, as cited by McDougall, *McDougall's Medicine*, p. 172.

[32] National Institutes of Health. "Diabetes Mellitus. Trans-NIH Research." NIH Pub No. 84-1982, May 1984, as cited by McDougall, *McDougall's Medicine*, p. 203.

[33] Winegrad A. Editorial: The complications of diabetes mellitus. N Engl J Med 298:1250, 1978, as cited by McDougall, *McDougall's Medicine*, p. 207.

[34] Kannel W. Diabetes and cardiovascular risk factors: the Farmingham study. Circulation 59:8, 1979. as cited by McDougall, *McDougall's Medicine*, p. 207.

[35] National Commission on Diabetes "The long-range plan to combat diabetes." Vol 1 DHEW Publication No (NIH) 76-1018, 1975, as cited by McDougall, *McDougall's Medicine*, p. 207.

[36] Cohen A. Myocardial infarction and carbohydrate metabolism. Geriatrics 23:158, 1968, as cited by McDougall, *McDougall's Medicine*, p. 207.

[37] McDougall, *McDougall's Medicine*, p. 237.

[38] Walker A. The human requirement of calcium: should low intakes be supplemented? Am J Clin Nutr 25:518, 1972, as cited by McDougall, *McDougall's Medicine*, p. 239.

[39] Lucas P. Dietary fat aggravates active rheumatoid arthritis. Clin Res 29:754A, 1981, as cited by McDougall, *McDougall's Medicine*, p. 243.

[40] Robertson W. Prevalence of urinary stone disease in vegetarians. Eur Urol 8:334, 1982, as cited by McDougall, *McDougall's Medicine*, p. 266.

[41] Whitaker, Julian. *The Prostate Report: Prevention and Healing* (Potomac, MD: Phillips Publishing, 1994), p. 38.

[42] Whitaker, p. 35.

[43] Whitaker, p. 36.

[44] Whitaker, p. 39.

[45] Whitaker, p. 29.

[46] Whitaker, p. 34.

[47] McDougall, *The McDougall Program*, p. 5.

[48] McDougall, *The McDougall Program* (cassette)

[49] Ley, Herbert, San Francisco Chronicle, January 2, 1970. Senator Edward Long, U. S. Senate hearings 1965, as cited by Lynes, Barry, *The Healing of Cancer* (Queensville, Ontario, Canada: Marcus Books, 1989), p. 17

Chapter 2

The Genesis Diet Heals

"My people perish for lack of knowledge" (Hosea 4:6)

We have discovered in Chapter One that the American diet is killing us, and that the initial diet that God gave us of high-fiber, low-fat and low-cholesterol, heals. I suppose that shouldn't come as a surprise. Jesus said that we can judge according to fruit. And obviously the fruit of the American diet is that the incidence of many degenerative diseases has been rising for many years.

Does the Bible Contain Answers to Society's Dilemmas?

When the bubonic plague was sweeping Europe and the medical community was helpless to stop it, some Christians got out their Bibles and re-discovered a truth buried in the depths of the Old Testament: that God had commanded the isolation of those with contagious diseases (Lev. 13:46). By practicing this long-lost and forgotten simple Old Testament command, they were able to stop the wholesale death of parents and children which was sweeping the land.

Maybe the Old Testament is not as outdated as we sometimes have thought it is. Perhaps since medical science is failing to find a cure for cancer, we should search Scriptures once again.

Why Did God Give the Genesis Diet?

"So God created man in his own image, in the image of God he created him; male and female he created them. God blessed them and said to them, 'Be fruitful and increase in number; fill the earth and subdue it. Rule over the fish of the sea and the birds of the air and over every living creature that moves on the ground.' Then God said, 'I give you every seed-bearing plant on the face of the whole earth and every tree that has fruit with seed in it. They will be yours for food. And to all the beasts of the earth and all the birds of the air and all the creatures that move on the ground — everything that has the breath of life in it —I give every green plant for food.' And it was so" (Gen. 2:27-31 NIV).

Here we have the first recorded words of God to man. He began with words of blessing, instruction and commission. "The earth is yours to fill and subdue and rule," He said. And to give them the strength to accomplish this mission, He then gave them a gift: "I give you every...plant...and every tree...for food" (Gen. 1:29 NIV). Sin had not yet entered the world, so there was no death (Rom. 6:23). Even the animals were vegetarians, living at peace with one another. Man's sin caused the first death of an animal, when God made garments of skin for Adam and Eve.

It is amazing to me how lightly I have considered these words of God in Genesis. Imagine the scene: God has created the earth and all the animals. He has established a special garden as a home for his crowning creation — man. He forms him from the dust of the ground and breathes into him the breath of life. Man awakens to the smiling face of his God. What will the Creator say? Will He waste time on small talk and unimportant chitchat? Of course not! He goes directly to essentials — "I want you and your family to take care of My earth and My creations and yourself. And this is how you take care of yourself — by eating these plants I have given you."

Why did God prescribe a specific diet to Adam and Eve? Why didn't He say, "Go, eat whatever you want"? Or, if our diet is as unimportant to God as we have chosen to believe it is, why did He bring up the subject at all?

I believe in a loving heavenly Father Who only gives commandments which are in my best interest, to grant me maximum life, joy, happiness, and peace. And that is what I believe about the Genesis diet. I believe God knew the best fuel for my body to run on and prescribed it to me. And our earliest ancestors did live more than 900 years on this diet. After the flood, God added meats and reduced man's life span to 120 years. I do suspect there were other reasons why people before the flood lived so long, but I cannot discount the possibility that the proper diet may have been one of the reasons. I am even more convinced when I read such books as *Become Younger* by Dr. N. W. Walker, who describes a lifestyle of living on a diet which is contained within the Genesis diet. He lived to 109 in vital health. By the way, I don't anticipate living to 900 now that I'm on the Genesis diet, but I do anticipate living to 100 or 120 in good health.

The Bible doesn't make it clear why God decided to add meats to mankind's diet. I find two verses which could possibly offer hints. One is Numbers 11:31 - 34 where we find that the Israelites begged Him for meat, and He sent it to them, and with it came leanness of soul (Psalm 106:15). Perhaps God was responding to man's **cravings and desires**.

A discussion between Jesus and the Pharisees in the New Testament may indicate that eating meat was God's **permissive will**, rather than His perfect will. In Matthew 19, when the Pharisees were testing Him, asking if it was lawful to divorce their wives, Jesus quoted Genesis 1:27 and 2:24, saying, "From the beginning it was not so, but Moses, **because of the hardness of your hearts** permitted you to divorce your wives." Perhaps God allowed meat for the same reason: because of the hardness of our hearts. From the beginning it was not so. Again, it is **not clear in Scriptures** why God allowed meat. These are **simply some suggestions**.

What Foods Does the Genesis Diet Include?

> "And God said, Behold, I have given you every herb bearing seed, which is upon the face of all the earth, and every tree, in the which is the fruit of a tree yielding seed; to you it shall be for meat." (Genesis 1:29 NASB)

It is probably easiest to define the above foods in terms of groupings to which we are accustomed. Starches, vegetables, fruits and nuts are the key categories of food in the Genesis diet. Starches, vegetables, and fruits are overlapping terms commonly applied to foods from the plant kingdom. They are generally poorly defined, even in our dictionaries, so we will use McDougall's definitions.

Starches: "Foods that contain adequate amounts of readily available calories in the form of starch molecules. Starch molecules are made of long chains of sugars, which are the basic units of our energy supply. These chains of sugars are accompanied by just the right amounts of protein, essential fat, fiber, water, vitamins and minerals. Starches are ideal foods around which to center your meal plan, and the starch foods should account for most of your daily calories."[1] A list of foods in this category can be found on the following pages.

Fruits: "Fruits contain most of their sugars in the simple form as sucrose, glucose, or fructose and therefore taste sweet. They yield plenty of calories and are generously supplied with fiber and vitamins. Most have adequate amounts of protein, minerals, and essential fat to be considered excellent, nutritionally complete foods."[2] A list of foods in this category is on the following pages.

"**Vegetables** will be defined as plants or plant parts that are too low in calorie content to form the center of a meal. However, they do provide valuable contributions of vitamins, minerals, fiber, water, essential fat, and protein...."[3] A list of foods in this category can be found on succeeding pages.

Nuts are an additional acceptable category in the Genesis diet.

The following diagrams show the various food groupings being recommended today. The American diet is what we have been taught in schools for the last 30 years or so. The Revised American diet can be found on ends of cereal boxes and other places and is the newest innovation. Both of these food groupings and diets have been promoted by the National Dairy Council, Kelloggs, Del Monte, Pillsbury, McDonald's or some other industrial interest.[4] They are not based in

The American Diet

A GUIDE TO GOOD EATING
Use Daily:

ADVERTISEMENT

MEAT GROUP
2 or more servings

MILK GROUP
3 or more servings

VEGETABLES AND FRUITS
4 or more servings

BREADS AND CEREALS
4 or more servings

Revised American Diet

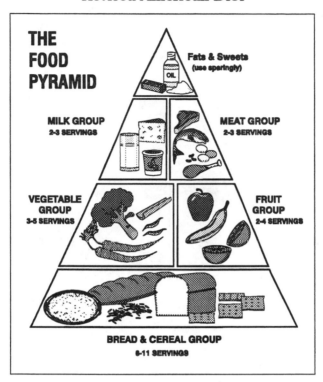

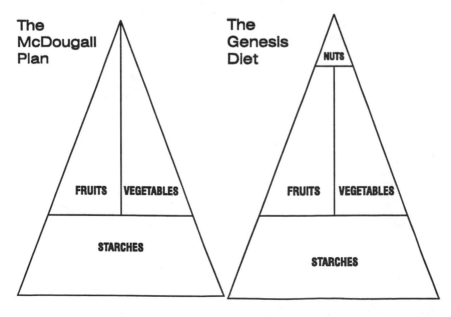

The Genesis Diet

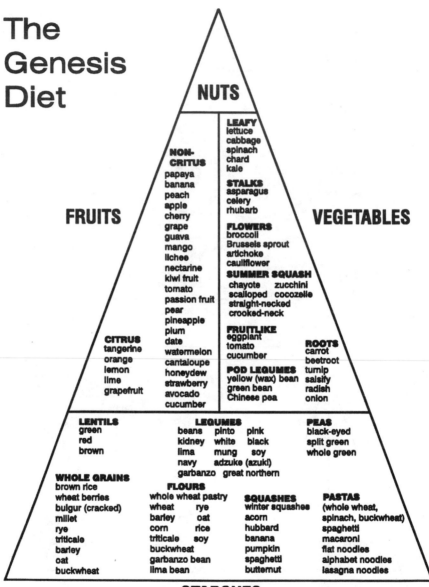

NUTS

FRUITS

VEGETABLES

NON-CRITUS
papaya
banana
peach
apple
cherry
grape
guava
mango
lichee
nectarine
kiwi fruit
tomato
passion fruit
pear
pineapple
plum
date
watermelon
cantaloupe
honeydew
strawberry
avocado
cucumber

CITRUS
tangerine
orange
lemon
lime
grapefruit

LEAFY
lettuce
cabbage
spinach
chard
kale

STALKS
asparagus
celery
rhubarb

FLOWERS
broccoli
Brussels sprout
artichoke
cauliflower

SUMMER SQUASH
chayote   zucchini
scalloped cocozelle
straight-necked
crooked-neck

FRUITLIKE
eggplant
tomato
cucumber

POD LEGUMES
yellow (wax) bean
green bean
Chinese pea

ROOTS
carrot
beetroot
turnip
salsify
radish
onion

LENTILS
green
red
brown

LEGUMES
beans   pinto   pink
kidney   white   black
lima   mung   soy
navy   adzuke (azuki)
garbanzo great northern

PEAS
black-eyed
split green
whole green

WHOLE GRAINS
brown rice
wheat berries
bulgur (cracked)
millet
rye
triticale
barley
oat
buckwheat

FLOURS
whole wheat pastry
wheat   rye
barley   oat
corn   rice
triticale   soy
buckwheat
garbanzo bean
lima bean

SQUASHES
winter squashes
acorn
hubbard
banana
pumpkin
spaghetti
butternut

PASTAS
(whole wheat,
spinach, buckwheat)
spaghetti
macaroni
flat noodles
alphabet noodles
lasagna noodles

STARCHES

scientific research, and do not promote health, as Chapter One made very obvious. They promote poor health, disease and early death. McDougall's books reference thousands of studies from all over the world which prove this. This is tragic because the unsuspecting American mom who has been trying her hardest to properly nourish her children has been led down the wrong path. Thank goodness our bodies begin to heal **the very same day** we alter our diets.

America didn't always have four food groups. There have been twelve food groups, then seven, then four, currently six. Dairy products and meats, and vegetables and fruit have sometimes been grouped together and sometimes separated. They are not at all the same, so maybe something is going on here which has nothing to do with enhancing health, life or vitality. I can find no reason to trust that the basic four food groups present any kind of a balanced healthy diet. They weren't the food groups God gave in the Genesis diet. I suspect the Genesis diet's food groups offer me a much more balanced diet than man's constantly-changing, politically-motivated, currently-listed six food groupings.

It doesn't bother me to adopt McDougall's diet, which does not include the nuts from the Genesis diet, because nuts are high in fat. Since my arteries and veins have so much cholesterol to lose before they are once again clean, I will go easy on the nuts. The triangular diagram of the food groups indicates that the majority of our diet should be starches, with fruits and vegetables in smaller amounts, and if you do include nuts, they should be very few.[5]

Righting the Imbalances

As you shift from the rich Western diet to the Genesis diet, you will be greatly reducing the amount of fat and cholesterol you take in and removing all animal protein. The shift will look something like this: (Fruits and vegetables have no cholesterol.)

	Genesis Diet	Rich Western Diet
Fat	5%	42%
Protein	10% (non-animal)	12% (much animal protein)
Carbohydrate	85%	46%
Total	100%	100%

Don't Eat the Fat

God very clearly commanded the Israelites not to eat the fat
(Lev. 3:17, 7:23,24).

> "It shall be a perpetual statute for your generations throughout all
> your dwellings, that ye eat neither fat nor blood" (Leviticus 3:17).

Not that they couldn't have a feast day and eat meat. That was
encouraged and even commanded (Neh. 8:10). However, we are not
designed to have 21 feast meals per week. You see, our bodies don't
process fat very well. It builds up in our blood and in our veins and
arteries. It has also been said that the fat you eat is the fat you wear.
Dr. Max Gerson suggests the following balance: three-quarters of the
food you eat should be taken for the purpose of nourishing your body's
basic systems; the remainder should be of your choice. That would
surely offer everyone plenty of freedom to choose his diet.

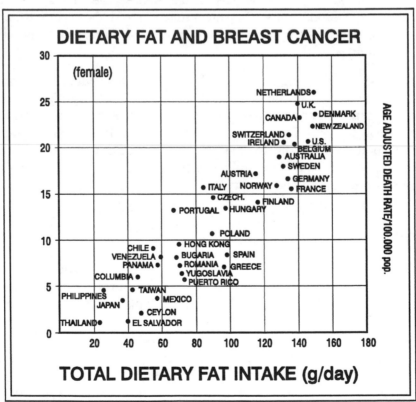

"Dietary fat consumption correlates most strongly with the risk of dying from
breast cancer in various countries."[7]

The diagram shows what happens when you consume a meal high in fat:

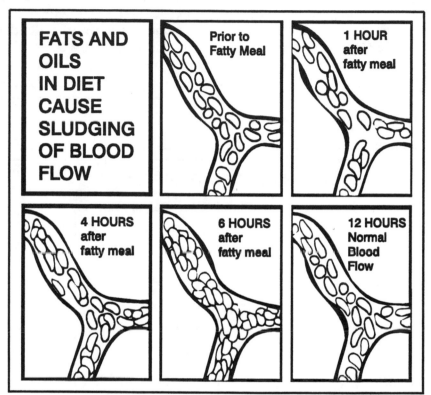

"Blood cells within a blood vessel flow freely and bounce off one another prior to a meal high in fat. Approximately one hour after a fatty meal, the cells begin to stick together upon contact and form small clumps. As this clump formation progresses, the flow of blood slows (sludging). Six hours after the meal the clumping becomes so severe that blood flow actually stops in some vessels. Several hours later the clumps break up and the blood flow returns to the tissue. Many people consume high-fat meals three and more times a day, causing continuous sludging of their blood, which in turn results in a poor supply of oxygen and other essential nutrients to their tissues all day long."[6]

This explains why so many Americans are sluggish after a meal: because approximately 20 percent of the oxygen supply to their bodies has been cut off for several hours. If you eat three high-fat meals per day, you are always running on 80 percent of the oxygen supply which God intended your body to run on (plus it is often polluted oxygen), and as your veins and arteries begin clogging, you have even less oxygen in your body. No wonder I was always tired. I feel so great and alive inside since I have switched to the Genesis diet and added a few herbs to my daily dietary intake! This is exciting because many great things happen within your body when you limit your fat consumption.

Other positive effects can occur when one consumes a low-fat diet like the Genesis diet, as opposed to the high-fat, rich Western diet. Cancers could be reduced to one-quarter the current rate, and sexual maturation could be put off in our young girls by three years. That, in itself, may be enough motivation for many Christian parents to put their families on the Genesis diet.

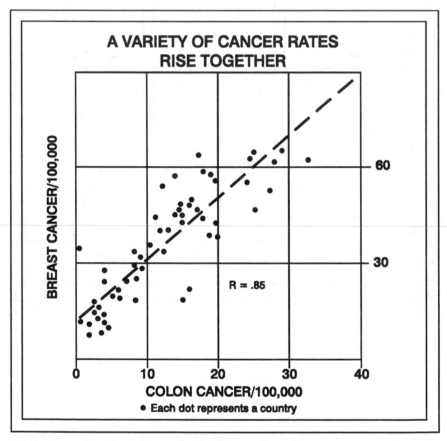

A VARIETY OF CANCER RATES RISE TOGETHER

BREAST CANCER/100,000

COLON CANCER/100,000

R = .85

• Each dot represents a country

"Because a rich diet is the causative factor shared by many types of cancer, people living in countries with high rates of one cancer usually have high rates of other cancers." [8]

A person eating the rich Western diet normally consumes about 140 grams of fat per day. If you use McDougall's diet and his cookbooks,

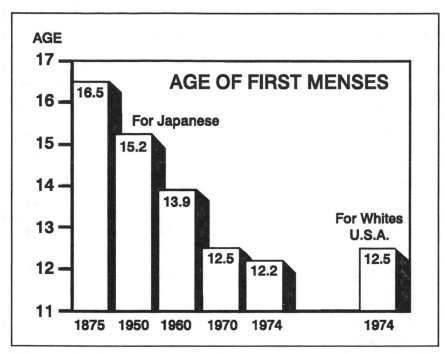

"Young girls in Japan are now maturing into women three years earlier than their ancestors because of a change from a traditional starch-centered diet of rice and vegetables to a richer fat-centered diet following World War II. Similar changes in maturation have taken place over the last century in most affluent western societies."[9]

as our family has begun to do, you will consume about 5 grams of fat per day. Incidentally, if you eat at Burger King, you can easily consume 100 grams of fat in a single meal. (That's equivalent to three weeks on the McDougall diet). The Burger King Double Whopper sandwich has 48 fat grams, medium fries have 20, and apple pie has 14, for a total so far of 82 fat grams, not counting your shake. When you eat at a salad bar, put a "no fat" dressing on your salad. A typical creamy Italian dressing has 7.1 grams of fat per tablespoon, but an Italian low-calorie dressing has only 1.5 grams of fat per tablespoon.

Other American institutions are beginning to move in the direction of God's commands. The American Heart Association, the American Cancer Society, and the American Diabetic Association all recommend eating less fat. However, none of them have yet come down to the amounts recommended by the Genesis diet. Oh, well. It takes man a long time to realize God was right all along.

OSTEOPOROSIS AND SELECTED NUTRIENTS [11-14]

Location	Hip fractures rate /100,000	Dairy intake grams/day/person	Protein intake grams/day/person	
			total	animal
United States	98	462	106	72
Sweden	70	502	89	59
Israel	59	315	105	57
Findland	44	711	93	61
United Kingdom	43	455	90	54
Hong Kong	32	95	82	50
Singapore	20	113	82	39
South Africa/ Black townships	6	10	55	11

Worldwide, the incidence of osteoporosis has a direct correlation to the total protein, and especially, the animal protein intake of a population of people; the more animal protein consumed by the people, the more the osteoporosis in the population. Furthermore, a high consumption of dairy product offers little protection for the bones, since countries with the highest intakes of these products— United States, Sweden, Israel, Finland, and the United Kingdom— also have the highest rates of osteoporosis-related hip fractures. Likewise, a low intake of dairy products appears to in no way harm the bones since the countries with the lowest intakes of dairy products—Hong King, Singapore, and rural Africa—have the lowest rates of osteoporosis. (All numbers have been rounded off to whole numbers. Figures for hip fractures from some countries may actually be from the population of a large city in that country.)

Categories of Food the Genesis Diet Omits

You may have noticed that the Genesis diet contains no meats or dairy products. These categories contain high fat and high cholesterol, and are extremely difficult for our bodies to effectively process. The number-two leading allergy in America is milk and dairy products, mainly because many people have an intolerance to lactose (i.e. milk sugar). About 40 million Americans have difficulty digesting lactose. We are not equipped to handle cow's milk. Yogurt does change the lactose so some, who just can't give up dairy products totally, might choose to use yogurt instead. In addition, yogurt is lower in fat than ice cream, and is rich in Lactobacillus acidophilus. (Check the label for live cultures.) Acidophilus is the friendly bacteria which populates one's intestines. A diet rich in meat destroys this bacteria. Yogurt helps replenish it.

The United States is the second largest consumer of dairy products in terms of grams per day per person. We also have the highest rate of hip fractures of any nation in the world. So contrary to the advertisements, milk does not give you strong bones. Cultures that consume a lot of dairy products **tend also to consume a lot of animal protein.**[10] Note the following chart on the following page.

Simply put, your body cannot store excess protein. Any extra protein which you eat in a day must be excreted, taking along many nutrients, including calcium. This in turn hollows out your bones, promoting osteoporosis. Your body can and will excrete **more** calcium on a diet high in animal protein than it is capable of re-absorbing through the digestive tract, so even supplements cannot **fully** offset the depletion of your bones if you are on a high animal-protein diet.

I have personally decreased my consumption of meat and dairy products by about 90 percent. I do not make a scene or offend my host if I am served these at a social gathering. Even the Bible says that there are feast days when we are to eat the fat (or rich foods, depending on the translation — Neh. 8:10). So I am not a strict vegetarian, but I have moved a long way in that direction.

Motivations for Relinquishing These Foods from Your Diet

There are several reasons it wasn't hard for me to give up meats or dairy products.

1. My doctor had informed me that I was moving rapidly toward a coronary problem. I did not want to die and leave my family when I was only in my forties. So, I was facing a crisis situation.

2. I had discovered a capsule with a combination of herbs and chromium which energized me, reduced my craving for food (including sweets), reduced the fat in my body, and increased my muscle. With my cravings gone and energy restored, I was once again ready to press on. (More detail on these herbs will be found in the chapter on herbs.) Since the herb/chromium combination removed my craving for food, I was able for the first time in my life to **view food sensibly rather than with insatiable desire**.

3. After reading McDougall's books, I became firmly convinced that meats and dairy products were poison to my system and were killing me. Once that **picture** was firmly planted in my mind, a deep aversion toward all meat and dairy products grew within me. You see, emotions are by-products of pictures in our minds. So, my new picture caused me to feel reluctant to eat meat. Others have shared with me that even though they loved meats and thought they could never give them up, they, too, found a distaste growing in them within just a few weeks.

4. I realized that most tastes are acquired. If I would give myself a few weeks, my taste buds would change, especially if I desired that and asked for God's assistance.

5. I realized that we have a natural aversion to meats. For example, if I were to tell you, "We have a great restaurant that serves horse and dog," you would be repulsed. If I can acquire a taste for something that initially is offensive to me, I can surely dis-acquire it.

6. We found three excellent recipe books by John and Mary McDougall with 500 recipes built around the Genesis diet. My wife has begun to cook from these and our entire family is growing to love them. I can highly recommend these books to you.

7. We found we were never hungry. We could eat all we wanted, even stuff ourselves, and still lose weight because we were eating the right kind of foods. Note the diagram below.

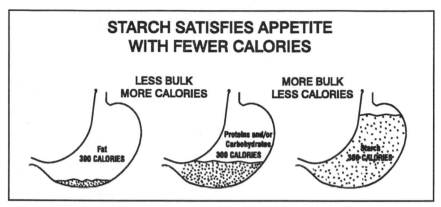

STARCH SATISFIES APPETITE
WITH FEWER CALORIES

"Hunger is satisfied by filling the stomach. Starches, vegetables, and fruits do this with fewer calories than meats, cheeses, and oils."[15]

Losing Weight on the Genesis Diet

Most people will lose weight on the Genesis diet, even though they eat all they want. To keep you from worrying about getting too thin, the following table from the Kempner Foundation may reassure you.[16]

WOMEN		MEN	
Height	**Weight** fully dressed [can safely go as low as] pounds:	**Height**	**Weight** fully dressed [can safely go as low as] pounds:
4'11"	91	5'2"	110
5'	94	5'3"	115
5'1"	97	5'4"	120
5'2"	100	5'5"	125
5'3"	104	5'6"	130
5'4"	108	5'7"	135
5'5"	112	5'8"	140
5'6"	117	5'9"	145
5'7"	122	5'10"	150
5'8"	127	5'11"	155
5'9"	132	6'	160
5'10"	137	6'1"	165
5'11"	142	6'2"	170
6'	147	6'3"	175
		6'4"	180
		6'5"	185

A Vegetarian Diet Increases Your Strength

Edwin Moses, an Olympic gold medalist who competed in the 400-meter hurdles for eight years without losing a single race, is a vegetarian. "Dave Scott, also a vegetarian, won the Hawaii Ironman Triatholon a record four times. He's recognized as the greatest triathlete in the world. In *Diet for a New America*, author John Robbins described several laboratory studies comparing meat eaters with vegetarians in strength and endurance. The results showed that vegetarians were two to three times stronger. **Stronger!** Imagine that!"[17] Does that remind you of Daniel?

Lowering Cholesterol and Blood Pressure on the Genesis Diet

In a study of 180 participants of the twelve-day live-in McDougall Program at St. Helena Hospital and Health Center, Napa Valley, CA, the average decrease in cholesterol was 28 mg/dl in twelve days and a corresponding 8 percent drop in blood pressure in the same twelve days with dietary changes only. At the same time, many of these people were coming off all their blood pressure medicine. They also lost two to seven pounds while eating all they could of the Genesis diet foods and never going hungry.[18]

Doesn't the Bible Allow Us to Eat Meats?

The fish that God permitted the Israelites to eat were the ones which have omega 3 oils, which are good for the heart. **However, moderation is essential.** Eskimos, who eat more fish than any other people in the world, also have the highest rate of osteoporosis of any people in the world.

Many people believe that the Bible presents three diets to us. One is the Genesis diet (the healthiest) found in Genesis 1. The second adds the clean meats, making it the next healthiest. The third includes the unclean meats, which is very unhealthy. God tells us four times in three verses that it is an **abomination** if we eat unclean fish (Lev. 11:10-12). I wonder if He thinks we are hard of hearing, or if He just knows that no matter how many times He says it, we will go ahead and eat them anyway. Guess what Americans eat: the un-healthiest of the three diets — the one that is an abomination — the unclean meats. If you want dietary evidence that the unclean meats are more damaging to your health than the clean meats, read *Clean and Unclean Foods* by Gordon Tessler, Ph.D.

Often believers try to prove from a few (misinterpreted) verses in the New Testament that God has changed His mind and we are now free to eat unclean meat. Rather than argue this point with you here, I prefer to refer the interested reader to two excellent books by Gordon Tessler entitled *Clean and Unclean Foods* and *Did God Change His Mind?* In the latter Tessler presents many pages of outstanding defense for interpreting the New Testament to show that God still did not allow unclean meat. Briefly stated, Tessler's defense includes:

1. Acts 10 — The vision of eating unclean animals, was **symbolism** and the Bible **clearly states the meaning** of the vision: God was showing Peter not to "call any man common or unclean" (Acts 10:28,29), and that he was to receive the Gentiles into the Church.

2. 1 Timothy 4:4 — "For every creature **of God** is good, and nothing is to be refused, if it be received with thanksgiving." What does "of God" mean? Does it mean all creatures are good to eat, or does it mean all creatures **of God** are good to eat? God talks about the children **of God** and the children **of the devil** (1 John 3:10). We must go to Scriptures to determine what is God's definition of a "child of God." So, too, we must go to Scripture to determine what God's definition is of a "creature of God." Scripture would define "a creature of God" as "a clean animal," as opposed to unclean animals. Or, if you go all the way back to the book of Genesis, the creatures (or foods) of God which were given to man to eat were the starches, fruits, vegetables and nuts.

    A second question you could ask concerning 1 Timothy 4:4 is, "What creatures can be received with thanksgiving?" Could we sincerely be thankful in our hearts before God for a meal of blood, fat, and other food that God has elsewhere warned us against? God is not changing the rules in this passage. He is saying that eating is not according to rules. It is according to relationship.

    The difference between the traditional Hebrew prayer said over a meal and the standard Christian prayer is striking.

    Hebrew prayer: "Blessed Art Thou, Oh Lord, our God, King of the Universe, who brings forth bread from the Earth."

    Christian prayer: "Bless this food to our bodies."

    A Jew never needs to ask God to bless the food he is about to eat, since the food is already sanctified by His Word, according to the Dietary Laws. Therefore, a Jew **blesses and thanks God** for the food he is about to eat. Since Christians tend to eat less than perfect food, we sense a need to ask God to bless it.

3.   Romans 14 — understood in the context of 1 Corinthians 8. Whenever we interpret Scriptures, we must put them in context. So let's try to get an understanding of Paul's beliefs and culture as we consider these passages. When Paul says "food" as an orthodox Jew, he is not thinking of unclean meats. Unclean meats are **not food** in Paul's mind. (If you say you are free to eat any meat you like, you probably are not trying to defend your lust for Morris, Lassie or Mr. Ed. Cat, dog and horse are **not food** to you.) So let's start interpreting these passages from **within the religious culture** of the one who wrote them, not from **our** definition of food. Some of us consider "junk food," which has almost no nutritional value, food. Biblically, food is nourishment. An orthodox Jew **never** considers unclean meats to be food. Some Corinthians wondered if they could eat food (i.e. clean animals) which had been offered to idols. Paul says it is acceptable, as long as you don't cause a fellow Christian to stumble (i.e. a Christian brother who is not sure if it is proper to eat food — clean meat — which has been offered to idols).

4.   1 Cor. 10:23 — "...all things are lawful for me" does not mean Paul can now go out and commit adultery. He means that even though the Old Testament law would allow him to eat clean meats offered to idols, he will not to so if it causes someone else to stumble.

5.   Matthew 15:11 — It is "not what goes into the mouth that defiles a man; but what comes out of the mouth, this defiles a man." (See also Mark 7:19 where it adds the phrase, "Thus He declared all foods clean".) The discussion here is not dietary law but what makes a person spiritually unclean. Jesus is saying is that the eating of various foods is not what contaminates one spiritually. Things like evil thoughts, fornications, thefts, murders, adulteries, and deeds of coveting are the spiritual contaminants (Mark 7:21-23).

For those wanting more extensive discussion of the these five points, I recommend a study of Tessler's books.

One vital point that should be screamed from the housetops is that I **do not believe** eating meats or some unclean meats will send you to hell. However, statistics indicate quite convincingly that it will get you to heaven sooner. I believe these are dietary laws, and you can choose the level of health and vitality you want to live in.

I do believe many of our prayers for healing have not been answered because we have not honored the Genesis diet. There is no record that Jesus ever healed cancer, high blood pressure, or coronary disease. Why not? I suspect it was because these problems did not exist for those Jews because they were eating a diet very different from ours.

Does a Partial Change in My Diet Help?

Change comes slowly for most of us, unless a traumatic situation forces a sudden turnaround. When I began my study on diet and nutrition, I remained on the diet I had always eaten, even though everything I was reading proved that it was killing me. When challenged on my inconsistency by my children, I responded, "I am in the process of building a spiritual conviction concerning food." And that was true. It takes time to build a spiritual conviction of sufficient depth to call one into a radically different lifestyle of eating. This is especially true in an area in which there is so much we have been taught that we need to unlearn. It is with reluctance that we accept the possibility that the health professionals, whom we have trusted, may have limitations in the advice which they offer because of their limited nutritional training and the impossible political climate in which they must work. Therefore, the development of new dietary convictions does not generally happen overnight.

So each of you will establish the pace and degree to which you will be changing your diet. I encourage you, for your own health's sake, to move at the fastest pace possible. The best way to speed up the change is to study and then experiment on your own body. The more I read and studied, the stronger and deeper my spiritual convictions grew, and the more I changed my diet, the better I felt.

Remember, any and every little dietary change in the right direction gives an immediate health benefit to your body. Even a one-quarter dietary change stimulates greatly improved health.

One Way to Increase the World Food Supply

Much more food can be given to many more people if we eat the Genesis diet. Consider the following. We get:

Product	Pounds / acre	Product	Pounds / acre
tomatoes	50,000	green beans	20,000
potatoes	40,000	beef	250
carrots	30,000		

Mentoring Assistance in Changing Your Diet

One company I work with offers a complete "Health Risk Appraisal" wherein a nurse does certain tests and measurements on your body and you answer a series of questions about your diet and lifestyle. The information received in this Appraisal is analyzed and a report returned to you. This report includes a specific personalized booklet showing your current health risks considering the way you are eating and living, along with specific recommendations of ways you could change that would add years to your life. Seeing your current health risks all charted on a graph can be good incentive for some to get them moving on the way to a healthier lifestyle. For those who want personal mentoring, this company also offers an on-line phone service which allows you to call a trained specialist who will help you find answers to the questions you have about the changes you are making. This company does not suggest the complete removal of meats and dairy products from your diet as we have in this chapter, but they do take many steps in the right direction. So this can be a "partial change" in diet, which may be more acceptable to some, and thus, easier to take while still being extremely valuable in improving your overall health.

Working Together as a Family

One can put 1000 to flight, and two 10,000 (Deut. 32:30). It is so much easier to be successful if the husband and wife both make this change together. I ask you to try it together for four weeks and just see what happens. I believe you will be so thrilled at the improvements in your health you will not go back to your old ways of eating.

Please, wives, do not feel attacked or condemned by what you have read in the last two chapters. Your goal has been to cook healthy food for your families, as an act of love and devotion to them. Now the suggestion is that the food may not actually have been the healthiest. I am in no way attacking your integrity or love or devotion toward your family. You have been doing the best you knew, according to the information we have all been given.

And, men, be the head in your families, and lead them into the ways of life. After all, they are your flock. Don't renege on your responsibility and allow the cravings of your flesh to rule your life and harm your family. Be men! Lead by your example.

At this point, God in His graciousness is restoring lost truths. When this happens, it is our responsibility to remain humble, non-defensive,

and pliable, as we embrace the things God is restoring. It is
been wrong. It happens to all of us all the time. Scriptures t
when we discover error, we are to repent and push on in new
That is what makes us different from stiff-necked Pharisees.
made the body with a wonderful capacity to heal itself if we simply give
it the chance. So I repent for my erroneous ways of eating and encourage others who need to, to do so, also. The vitality and life you
experience in the first four weeks on the Genesis diet will bless your
heart and life.

Additional Reading

The McDougall Health-Supporting Cookbooks Volumes I & II. Each
volume contains 250 original delicious recipes built around the Genesis
diet.

Clean and Unclean Foods by Gordon Tessler. A study of the dietary and
health reasons why God permitted us to eat certain animals and not
others.

Did God Change His Mind? by Gordon Tessler. A study of about half a
dozen key New Testament references which seem to indicate that God
has changed His mind and we can now eat unclean meat. Tessler shows
that this is not what these passages are saying.

Other books of interest

The following three books are by Norman Walker. They were written
20 to 50 years ago, so they could seem a bit dated. Dr. Walker is
extremely conservative in his approach to eating, more than many will
choose to be. However, if you want to go "all the way," he probably
describes "all the way" as well as anyone! Patti and I are personally a
bit more moderate than Dr. Walker, although if fighting to overcome a
major disease, Dr. Walker and Dr. Gerson list the diet we would go on.

Become Younger by Dr. N.W. Walker. An outstanding 120 pages over-
viewing steps to longevity. Dr. Walker lived in vital health to 109, dying
in 1985. In one of his many books, he observed that "while such food
[dead, processed food] can, and does, sustain life in the human system,
it does so at the expense of progressively degenerating health, energy,
and vitality."

Natural Weight Control by Norman W. Walker. How eating right causes
you to maintain your weight.

The Natural Way to Vibrant Health by Dr. N.W. Walker

The Back to Eden Cookbook by Jethro Kloss. Health-oriented recipes.

The Food Pharmacy by Jean Carper. How to choose the right food to fight various diseases.

References

[1] McDougall, John, *The McDougall Plan* (Clinton, NJ: New Win Publishing, 1983), p. 30.

[2] McDougall, p. 31.

[3] McDougall, p. 32.

[4] McDougall, p. 2.

[5] McDougall, pp. 30 - 33.

[6] McDougall, p. 79.

[7] K. Carroll, *Cancer Res* 35 (1975):3374, as cited by McDougall, p. 83.

[8] A. Lowenfels, *Cancer 39* (1977):1809, as cited by McDougall, p. 84.

[9] Y. Kagawa, *Prev Med* 7 (1978):205, as cited by McDougall, p. 87.

[10] See McDougall, John, *McDougall's Medicine: A Challenging Second Opinion* (Clinton, NJ: New Win Publishing, 1985), pp. 67 - 80.

[11] Walker A. The human requirement of calcium: should low intakes be supplemented? Am J Clin Nutr 25:518, 1972, as cited by McDougall, *McDougall's Medicine*, p. 68.

[12] Lewinnek G. The significance and a comparative analysis of the epideiology of hip fractures. Clin Ortho Related Res 152:35, 1980, as cited by McDougall, *McDougall's Medicine*, p. 68.

[13] Food balance sheets. 1979-1981 average. Food and Agriculture Organization of the United Nations. Rome. 1984, as cited by McDougall, *McDougall's Medicine*, p. 68.

[14] *FAO production yearbook*. 37:263, 1984, as cited by McDougall, *McDougall's Medicine*, p. 68.

[15] McDougall, *The McDougall Plan*, p. 23.

[16] McDougall, *The McDougall Plan*, p. 28.

[17] Frahm, Anne with David J. Frahm. *A Cancer Battle Plan* (Colorado Springs, CO: Pinon Press, 1992), p. 75.

[18] McDougall, *The McDougall Program* (New York: Penguin Books, 1990) pp. 28, 29.

Chapter 3

Understanding How Our Bodies Fight Disease

Central to our understanding of how to live free of disease, and how to be healed, is to understand what disease is and how marvelously God has created the human body to conduct its own high-tech ballistic warfare using specialized smart missiles which it creates itself. These weapons are specifically designed to effectively demolish any and every bacterial invasion and mutated cell. All foreign bacteria and mutated cells are viewed as toxic by the body's immune system. The immune system fights to remove these toxic cells, thus detoxifying the body. It is high-tech warfare of the most amazing kind, and it is taking place continuously within your body. As long as you give your body the proper nourishment with which to create these smart missiles, **and** you limit the number of mutated cells or foreign bacteria which you allow into your body, your inner defense system will be victorious in its efforts and you will stay healthy.

A Holistic Approach to Treating Cancer

Max Gerson M.D., author of *A Cancer Therapy: Results of Fifty Cases* and *The Cure of Advanced Cancer by Diet Therapy*, states: "The treatment [of cancer] has to fulfill two fundamental components. The first component is the detoxification of the whole body which has to be carried out over a long period of time, until all the tumors are absorbed and the essential organs of the body are so far restored that they can take over this important 'cleaning function' by themselves....Secondly, the entire intestinal tract has to be restored simultaneously....In that way we can activate, together with other functions, defense, immunity and healing power in the body....For that purpose, the degree of restoration of the liver plays a decisive role."[1]

Understanding the Lymphatic System's Fight Against Mutated Cells

God has designed the body's cellular system with unbelievable intricacy. It is still very poorly understood and seldom fully appreciated. First of all, most of the cells in the body are constantly being replaced through a growth and division process. Every year you receive an almost entirely new body. How is that for rejuvenation! That means if you take good care of your body's needs for a year, you can have a much improved body at the end of that year!

The body's cells are surrounded by tissue fluid which provides a proper balance of water and electrolyte concentration. It is this tissue fluid which acts as the battlefield in which your body fights off invading microorganisms. The lymphatic system works as a drainage and sanitation system for tissue fluid, which is called lymph once it enters lymph vessels. The lymph system is a one-way transportation system and does not circulate like the blood. It has no pump to move the lymph along and therefore it relies on bodily movement to propel it. Just about anything that compresses the lymph vessel can also cause pumping, such as the contraction of a muscle, arterial pulsations, and even a body massage. However, the movement of skeletal muscles is the major force that moves lymph. During exercise, the lymph flow is increased 10 to 30 fold. That is one reason why exercise is so healing to the body, and reduces the body's susceptibility to **all disease** by 30 percent. A body without movement is like a nation at war that cannot move its army to the battlefields. If you feel like you are "coming down with something," vigorous exercise could do wonders to speed your immune system's strategic fighters to the battle site.

Special white blood cells called lymphocytes are produced in the bone marrow. Before they reach full maturity, about half find their way to the thymus where they develop into T-lymphocytes. The rest become B-lymphocytes in the bones. Both types circulate in the blood and many settle in the lymph nodes, available for instant action in case of an invasion. T-lymphocytes may destroy enemy cells by phagocytosis (ingesting them like little "Pac-men") or by injecting a poison such as hydrogen peroxide into them. B-lymphocytes are able to produce a massive army of antibodies when a particular foreign substance is identified in the body. Antibodies are small molecules that scurry around checking the identification of every cell in the entire body. Other cells which work tirelessly to keep you healthy include neutrophils, leukocytes and monocytes, which develop into macrophages.

Each molecule of your body carries an identification message known as an epitope, which consists of about ten "letters" made up of amino acids. These "badges" stick out from each molecule and are challenged by any antibody that comes near it. If an antibody discovers that a molecule is a foreigner, it immediately attaches itself to the invader and sends a signal to other antibodies, T-lymphocytes and neutrophils, which all proceed as fast as possible from all directions to the site of the antibody arrest. There is no judge or jury. The fact that the cell carries the wrong information on its epitope is proof enough, and it is immediately destroyed. T-cells have the ability to put another hundred lymphocytes in the area on alert. In turn, each of the hundred lymphos who answer the call also has the ability to recruit hundreds more.

If the lymphatic system is strong, healthy, circulating properly, and kept well-informed by the antibodies, the lymphocytes can get in there and clean up problems in no time flat. But, if the crack armies of your immune defense forces are weakened by lack of proper exercise, imperfect nutrition, or the presence of too much toxic waste in the body, the balance of power can swing in favor of the mutant cells. Then the mutants develop a law unto themselves and build a cancer colony.

The Origin of Cancer Cells

A cell must mutate twice before it becomes a cancer cell. In every instance, a cancer cell is caused by mutations of the genes in the DNA that control **both** cell growth and cell reproduction. It then develops into a colony that grows unchecked. This sequence is kept at bay because 1) most cell mutations have less survival capability than normal cells; 2) only a few mutated cells actually disobey the normal feedback controls that prevent excessive growth; and 3) the cells that are potentially cancerous are the target of search and destroy teams of one's immune system, and they are cleaned out long before they form into a cancer colony. Our bodies have cancerous cells (mutated cells) within them all the time. However, they are constantly being cleaned out by an effective immune system before they grow into a colony. Only about one out of every thousand cancer cells can survive more than two weeks. Most of us never know about 95 percent of the cancer colonies in our bodies. The only ones we know about are the ones which overwhelm the immune defense forces.

So actually, nothing causes cancer, but an inefficient immune system allows cancer to develop. *The American Cancer Society Cancer Book* reads, "Only when the immune system is incapable of destroying these malignant cells will cancer develop" (page XIX 1986 edition). Cancer is not a disease. It is a symptom of an inefficient immune system, and a signal to you to detoxify your body and build your immune system.

Unbelievable! So the cure for cancer is to make sure the immune system is strong and active, and it will send internal missiles to kill off any and all cancer cells. No wonder it has taken medical scientists so long to discover the cancer virus. THERE ISN'T ONE! The break-through in cancer will come in the strengthening of the immune system. The rest of the chapters of this book are devoted to both the strengthening of the immune system and the reduction of poisonous chemicals which are allowed to infiltrate the body.

Unfortunately, the traditional cancer therapies of radiation and chemotherapy not only destroy the cancer colonies, they also annihilate the antibodies and macrophages and T-lymphocytes which are surrounding, fighting and destroying the cancer colonies. In addition, radiation produces more mutated cells which can easily become cancerous themselves. It seems to me that rather than using external poisonous missiles which destroy both the good and the bad cells, it would be better to nourish and strengthen your body's own natural defense ballistic missile system which accurately identifies every mutant cell and devours only those bad cells, leaving all good cells untouched.

Cancer signals a breakdown of the immune system. To fight it, let's strengthen the immune system, not destroy it even more. Rather than cut and mutilate the body, let's arm the inner warheads and increase their production through proper nourishment, sending them out with greater speed through a little exercise. There is so much we can do **working within** our natural defense system, rather than wreaking havoc on it from outside.

And have you noticed that medical authorities have decided that various key parts of the body's lymphatic system are not really necessary and they often cut them out? This includes the tonsils and adenoids, the lymph nodes, the appendix and the spleen. Say good-bye to your immune system. A bit scary, isn't it?

By the way, before scientists can conduct experiments on mice to find new ways of externally poisoning the mouse's mutated (cancerous) cells, they must first breed a strain of mice which has no immune system. (We can't have the body's natural defense system messing up our experiments and healing itself naturally!)

Cancer Signals a Breakdown of the Body's Immune System

Dr. Max Gerson puts it this way. "Cancer is an extraordinary symptom only. The underlying cause is to be found in the poisoning of the liver."[2] He continues:

> "After more than 25 years of cancer work I can draw the following conclusions:
>
> 1) Cancer is not a local but a general disease, caused chiefly by the poisoning of foodstuffs prepared by modern farming and food industry. Medicine must be able to adapt its therapeutic methods to the damages of the processes of our modern civilization.
>
> 2) A method is elaborated to detoxify the body, kill the tumor masses and to absorb and eliminate them. (Restoration of the healing power.)
>
> 3) A way has been found to restore the liver if not too far destroyed and repair the destruction caused by the tumor masses.
>
> 4) To prove the return of the allergic reaction (healing power), cantharidin plasters are applied on the skin at weekly or longer intervals."[3]

Now let me repeat what I said in the first chapter. It is so important that I want to say it over and over again. **The bottom line** is that degenerative diseases (and the aging process itself) can be slowed, halted, and even reversed by doing three simple things:

1) detoxifying the body;
2) strengthening the immune system; and
3) nourishing your cells.

This is true because the growth of mutated cells causes degenerative diseases (cancer, etc.) and the aging process. A strong lymphatic system (immune system) eats up and destroys mutated cells before they can multiply into growths, diseases and aging symptoms. Healthy nourishment provides you with a healthy immune system and a healthy body.

Therefore, everything we study in this book heals by doing at least one of three things: 1) It detoxifies the body; 2) It builds the immune system;

or 3) It nourishes the body. Be constantly aware of how you are doing these things, and God's covenant of health will be yours (Ex. 15:26).

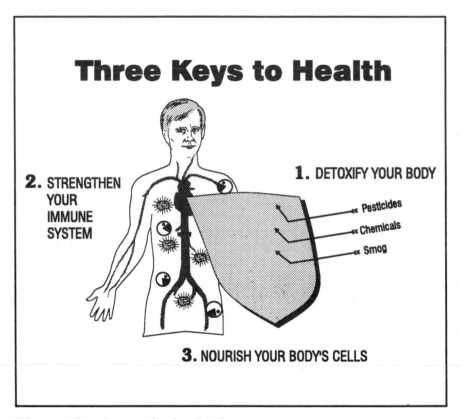

Three Keys to Health

2. STRENGTHEN YOUR IMMUNE SYSTEM

1. DETOXIFY YOUR BODY

« Pesticides

« Chemicals

« Smog

3. NOURISH YOUR BODY'S CELLS

Things That Detoxify the Body:
* Eating the Genesis diet
* Breathing pure air
* Drinking pure water
* Eating pure, vital food
* Excreting waste from the intestines quickly
* Using herbs wisely
* Super-foods
* taking vitamins and minerials
* Removing toxic chemicals from surfaces which one touches
* Taking antioxidants
* Fasting
* Prayer for healing.

Things Which Strengthen the Immune System:
* Eating the Genesis diet
* Prayer for healing
* Being healed of past emotional traumas
* Living in a spirit of faith, hope and love
* Eating pure, vital food
* exercising
* Taking vitamins and minerals
* Using herbs wisely
* Taking aloe vera
* Pycnogenol
* DHEA
* Superfoods
* Co-enzyme Q10.

Things Which Nourish the Cells:
* Eating the Genesis diet
* Super-foods
* Breathing pure air
* Taking vitamins and minerals
* Drinking lots of pure water
* Co-enzyme Q10.

A Healthy Immune System Versus an Unhealthy Immune System

Dr. Max Gerson lists six steps in the development of cancer (and/or degenerative diseases in general).

LIFE MEANS:	CANCER MEANS:
1. Maintenance of the normal metabolism, its regulations and productions of hormones, enzymes, co-enzymes, etc., absorption and elimination power.	1. Slow intoxication and alteration of the whole body, especially the liver.

2. Maintaining the prevalence of the potassium [K] group in vital organs and Na-group [sodium] mainly outside in the fluids and some tissues.

2. Invasion of the Na-group [sodium], loss of K-group [potassium], followed by tissue edema.

3. Keeping the positive electrical potentials of the cells high as the basis for energy and function, simultaneously as a defense against invasion of the Na-group and the formation of edema.

3. Lower electrical potentials in vital organs, more edema, accumulation of poisons, loss of tension, tonus, reduced re-activation and oxidation power, dedifferentiation of some cells.

4. Maintenance of circulation, tension, tonus, storage capacity, reserves.

4. Cancer starts — general poisoning increases, vital functions and energies decrease — cancer increases.

5. Re-activation power of vital substances, especially enzymes.

5. Further destruction of the metabolism and liver parenchym — cancer rules — is acting, spreading.

6. Defense and healing power.

6. Loss of last defense — hepatic coma — death."[4]

If the above chart loses you a bit, especially in the discussion of the potassium group versus sodium group, let me explain. Some diets we may eat have a much higher potassium (K) content, and some a much higher sodium content (Na). The breakdown is as follows:

	Genesis Diet	**Rich Western Diet**
Sodium (Na)	1000 mg	5000 mg
Potassium (K)	5000 mg	2000 mg

Cancer cells grow when sodium and potassium are not kept in proper balance in one's body. Health flourishes and is restored when the proper balance is restored. The Genesis diet restores the proper balance. The Genesis diet heals!

Studies have shown that people who eat lots of good, fresh, unprocessed fruits and vegetables and steer clear of red meats have much lower risks of major life-threatening diseases. For example, a recent review of 170 studies from seventeen nations revealed that people who eat the most fruits and vegetables consistently have half the cancer rates of those who eat the least. That includes cancers of the lung, colon, breast, cervix, esophagus, stomach, bladder, pancreas and ovary. Research also shows that eating vegetables twice a day cuts the risk of lung cancer by 50 percent, even in ex-smokers. Perhaps most exciting of all is new research at Tufts University that shows that beta carotene can actually change in the body to retinoic acid, a substance used to treat certain cancers. And beta carotene is just one cancer-fighting chemical concentrated in vegetables and fruits.[5]

For Further Reading

Biology, God's Living Creation by Keith Graham, Laurel Hicks, Delores Shimmin, George Thompson. A Beka Book. Especially pages 306-319 give an overview of the lymph system.

A Cancer Therapy & The Cure of Advanced Cancer by Diet Therapy by Max Gerson, M.D. A scholarly book with a healing diet detailed. One is allowed to eat a selected portion of the Genesis diet, under strict guidelines. I would follow this if I had cancer.

The Cancer Answer by Albert Earl Carter & Larry Lymphocyte. This book makes a wonderful companion to the above book by Max Gerson. Max Gerson will give you a scientific overview and Albert Carter carries on an imaginary conversation with one of his Lymphocytes (Larry Lymphocyte) concerning the application of the truths of Max Gerson's book. Together they form a grand pair of books! This book will change you forever and give you absolutely clear answers as to what cancer is and how to heal it yourself.

Cancer Battle Plan by Anne E. Frahm. An excellent story and teaching of how to beat cancer using alternative medicine. Anne spent one-and-a-half years being cut, mutilated and radiated by the medical community and was then sent home to die. Back home she went on a nutritional diet and was freed of all cancer within six weeks. I would follow its guidelines if I had cancer.

Cancer and Vitamin C by Ewan Cameron and Linus Pauling. Contains 270 pages of research results on how mega doses of vitamin C (and other antioxidants) can effectively stop cancer. If I had cancer I would be taking their recommended doses of vitamins which they have proven retard cancer growth and even throw it into remission. The following is a quote from their book: "It is accordingly our strong recommendation that every patient with cancer begin, as early in the course of the disease as possible, to follow the nutritional regimen advocated by Dr. Hoffer. This regimen involves a daily intake of about 12,000 mg of vitamin C, 800 IU of vitamin E, 1,500 mg of niacin (vitamin B3, either nicotinic acid or nicotinamide), 25 or 50 times the RDA of other B vitamins, 0.200 mg of selenium, and for some patients supplementary amounts of other minerals, such as zinc or calcium."[6]

References

[1] Gerson, Max, *A Cancer Therapy* (Bonita, CA: The Gerson Institute, 1990), pp. 16,17.

[2] Gerson, p. 165.

[3] Gerson, p. 199.

[4] Gerson, p. 102.

[5] "Ladies' Home Journal," August 1993, pp. 82,84.

[6] Cameron, Ewan, and Linus Pauling, *Cancer and Vitamin C* (Philadelphia, PA: Camino Books, 1979, 1993), p. xxiii.

Chapter 4

Recovering Living Land and Living Food

In the Garden of Eden, the land was pure, the air was pure, the water was pure, and the diet was wholesome. In that environment, people lived 900 years and more. When man sinned, pollution of every kind entered the world. Man no longer knew how to relate to his fellow man, the earth, or the creatures of the world as God intended. Sin, sickness and death filled the earth.

But God called forth a nation to be His own, to be different, set apart, sanctified, holy, clean. Because of sin, He couldn't simply place them in the land which He had prepared for them and expect them to live His way. He therefore gave them instructions to guide every aspect of their lives. Every guideline or law was designed to enhance the quality of their lives. No law was given lightly or for petty authoritarian purposes. Every line and precept was for blessing and provision, to restore to them the vitality of the Garden of Eden where man walked and talked with God in holiness in the cool of the day. These laws not only were to make their physical lives better, they governed their relationship to God. And the spirit of the laws God gave is purity (Lev. 19:2;20:7,26). Leviticus speaks of clean versus unclean, pure versus defiled, and holy versus common.

Most people would agree it is wise to provide our bodies with the purest water, purest air and purest food we possibly can. I believe our bodies will operate best in this environment. Obviously, the more air, food, and water we consume which is contaminated with pollutants, the more our bodies must struggle to cleanse out mutated cells which become damaged by these pollutants. When we take in a heavy load of toxins through food, water, and air, we put an excessive cleansing responsibility on our bodies' immune system, which is responsible to keep our insides free of damaged and mutated cells before they begin multiplying. The immune system can become overwhelmed, allowing cancer or other degenerative diseases to develop. Or, our immune system can break down, and environmental sickness can be the result. Therefore, anything we can do to reduce the load of toxins we take in will ultimately improve our health.

It is pretty well accepted in America that the toxic chemicals in cigarette smoke pollute our bodies with chemical poisons and cause them to break down with cancer. It is for the same reason that we also avoid many other toxic chemicals. Let's apply the **spirit of the laws** of Leviticus (i.e. the laws of purity) to our modern lifestyle.

Let's assume we start with the right kind of food

We will assume you are planning to make the change from the rich Western diet to the Genesis diet. You are going to take a stand like Daniel, who "made up his mind that he would not defile himself with the king's choice food or with the wine which he drank" (Dan. 1:8) and chose instead to live on vegetables and water (Dan. 1:12).

What do I need to be aware of that can contaminate even the Genesis foods? There are several possibilities.

Depleted soil

Dr. Max Gerson states: "The damage that modern civilization brings into our lives begins with the soil, where artificial fertilization leads to the displacement of mineral contents and changes in the flora of microbes combined with the exodus of the earthworms."[1]

Dr. Gerson's book entitled *A Cancer Therapy* gives the results of tests which show what happens to the soil when it is cropped year after year and not allowed to lie fallow every seventh year as the Lord commanded.[2] According to the study Dr. Gerson quotes, the average composition of soil was as follows:

1. Land which had had crops on it for eight years was composed of 1,097 parts per million of nutritional solids.
2. Land left fallow for eight years was 2,871 parts per million of nutritional solids.

"But in the seventh year shall be a sabbath of rest unto the land, a sabbath for the LORD: thou shalt neither sow thy field, nor prune thy vineyard." (Leviticus 25:4)

Central to Dr. Gerson's treatment of cancer is that patients drink large quantities of freshly-made fruit juices. The necessary fruit is specially grown and the juices made at his institute. After a number of years of treating his cancer patients with the juices, the healing effects of his regimen began to diminish. When he tested his juices for nutritional value, he found they had become immensely devalued over the years because of poor farming techniques.

This helps explain why the nutritional advice we were given by our mothers may not be as accurate today as it was when they learned it. The land and the food of today are very different from those of only forty years ago.

God designed the land to LIVE!

Several months ago I was privileged to meet Albert I. Ocker, a Christian consultant to farmers and gardeners and a man who has given the last forty-four years of his life to the study of the land. Since I was raised on a farm and grew up with a love of the land, I thoroughly enjoyed the hours spent one evening, listening to him share his revelations concerning the land. That which follows comes from those discussions as well as the books he lent me.

God's design for the land was that it was to **replenish itself** naturally through the micro-organizations which He placed in it. The land was literally alive and teaming with life, which would decompose plants and replenish the soil.

"And God said, **Let the earth bring forth** grass, the herb yielding seed, and the fruit tree yielding fruit after his kind, whose seed is in itself, upon the earth: and it was so. **And the earth brought forth** grass, and herb yielding seed after his kind, and the tree yielding fruit, whose seed was in itself, after his kind: and God saw that it was good" (Genesis 1:11-12).

"Microbes require a delicate balance of soil in order to live and survive. An ideal condition would provide for 5% humus, 45% mineral, 25% air and 25% water....The term 'microorganism' covers a broad array of living organisms including bacteria, actinomycetes, fungi, algae, protozoa, and nematodes. These decomposers play the crucial role of breaking down organic waste into usable nutrients which are then chelated or locked into the resulting 'humus'."[3]

Fertilized land becomes compacted and dead

Around 1945, agricultural "experts" decided that the earth needed help in bringing forth crops, and the use of chemical fertilizers began. Unfortunately, the very chemicals applied cause the millions of micro-organisms which God has placed in the ground, which made it "living land", to flee, and so the ground became quite sterile. It has been called dead land, biologically speaking. Much of North American soil which has been intensely farmed consists of dead land.

Plant life grown in dead land becomes very sickly. Phillip Callahan has recorded studies in his books (*Turning into Nature* and *The Sound of the Ghost Moth*) showing that insects will attack unhealthy plants, leaving healthy plants alone. The farmer now has the problem of insects destroying his unhealthy crop, so he must spray with poisons to kill the insects. We, the consumers, then eat the plant with the poison on it and very little nutritional value in it. These poisons, of course, find their way through our bodies, causing destruction on the molecular level which must be cleaned up by our immune system, or the damaged cells will contribute to various degenerative diseases.

Compacted soil yields less crops

Once most of the microbes and fishworms are out of the soil, soil compaction sets in and water tends to run off the land rather than soak into it, and the crops decrease. A "penetrometer" is an instrument which will measure the amount of soil compaction that has actually taken place.

Purdue University experiments on silt loam soils proved that both moderate and severe compaction of the subsoil: 1) reduce corn plant height; 2) increase moisture content at harvest; and 3) reduce yields. Details are shown in the charts on the following page.[4]

Ohio scientists reported a 30 percent reduction in corn yields when soil was compacted at the three to six inch depth. Illinois scientists reported twelve bushels less per acre from compaction of a silty clay-loam soil. Also in Illinois, Elanco Products Company researchers demonstrated a 60 percent yield reduction — from 159 bushels to only 96 bushels — due to compaction.

Solutions are available. For instance, a farmer can purchase equipment called an AerWay which "shatters" the land, breaking up the compacted soil.

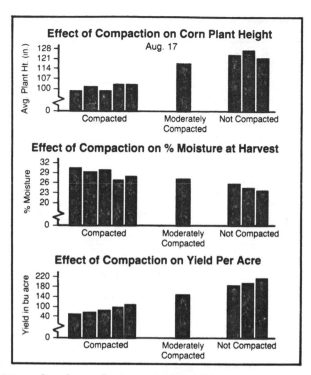

The nutritional value of crops is less from compacted soil

Even more serious than lower production is the loss of nutritional content in the food from chemically treated land. A refractometer, a simple hand-held instrument which can be purchased for about $230, measures the dissolved sugars (brix) present in a plant or vegetable. It consists of a tube shaped instrument with an adjustable eyepiece at one end and a prism with a plastic cover at the other end. Brix are a measure of the health of the plant and its nutritional value to you. By placing a drop of plant juice on the refractometer, you can get an accurate reading of the nutritional value of any plant food.

Following is a refractive index of crop juices calibrated in "o brix". According to Mr. Ocker, you would probably find that the foods in today's supermarkets are off the low end of the scale, and thus have value only to SUSTAIN life within your cells and not NOURISH life.

No quality control on nutritional content

Today, it is virtually impossible to purchase Genesis food which has in it all the goodness which God intended it to have. Therefore, even though I am eating right, I want to supplement my diet with vitamins and other health products.

Fruits	Poor	Excellent	Vegetables	Poor	Excellent
Apples	6	18	Asparagus	2	8
Avocados	4	10	Beets	2	12
Bananas	8	14	Bell Peppers	4	12
Cantaloupe	8	16	Broccoli	6	12
Casaba	8	14	Cabbage	6	12
Cherries, sweet	6	26	Carrots	6	18
Cherries, tart	6	18	Cauliflower	4	10
Coconut	8	14	Celery	4	12
Grapes	8	24	Corn Stalks	4	20
Grapefruit	6	18	Field Corn	6	18
Honeydew	8	14	Sweet Corn	6	24
Kumquat	4	10	Cow Peas	4	12
Lemons	4	12	Endive	4	10
Limes	4	12	English Peas	4	10
Mangoes	4	14	Escarole	4	10
Oranges	6	20	Field Peas	4	12
Papayas	6	22	Green Beans	4	10
Peaches	6	18	Hot Peppers	4	10
Pears	6	14	Kohlrabi	6	12
Pineapple	12	22	Lettuce	4	10
Raisins	60	80	Onions	4	10
Raspberries	6	14	Parsley	4	10
Strawberries	6	16	Peanuts	4	10
Watermelon	8	16	Potatoes, Irish	3	7
Grasses			Potatoes, Red	3	7
Alfalfa	4	22	Potatoes, Sweet	6	14
Cotton	4	22	Romaine	4	10
Grains	6	18	Rutabagas	4	12
Rice	4	16	Squash	6	12
Soybeans	4	16	Sorghum	6	30
Turnips	4	10	Tomatoes	4	12 [5]

A case in point: The nutrient content of cattle forage has been tested for years because dairy farmers won't buy a load of hay unless it meets their strict nutrient requirements. A recent study of cattle forage testing revealed that concentrations of calcium in cattle forage plants varied 568 percent, depending on the field in which it was grown. The study showed a 292 percent difference in phosphorus content, 450 percent in cobalt, 400 percent in copper, 740 percent in manganese and 260 percent in zinc.

So who is testing our food for vitamin and mineral content? NO ONE! No law requires any level of nutritional value. No inspector checks for nutritional value. We care more about the nutritional value of the hay we feed our cattle than the food we put in our mouths. Perhaps that is one reason Americans are so sickly and feel such low energy.

What Is in the Foods We Eat?

Let's do an experiment with a couple of foods which you may currently purchase off a grocery store shelf in the U.S. One we will call Product A, the other Product B. When you read the label on a product, whatever there is the most of appears first, and then the rest of the ingredients are listed in descending order.

Product A
1. Whole grain wheat
2. Sugar
3. Whole grain brown rice
4. Tricalcium & dicalcium phosphate
5. Salt
6. Malt extract
7. Corn syrup (sugar)
8. BHT
9. Several vitamins & minerals

Product B
1. Wheat flour
2. Soybean meal
3. Meat and bone meal
4. Whole milk
5. Wheat germ
6. Whole wheat
7. Salt
8. Calcium
9. Fish meal
10. Corn
11. Brewers yeast
12. Yeast extract
13. Molasses (sugar)
14. Several vitamins
    and minerals

From a nutritional standpoint, would you say that Product A is the superior product or Product B? Product A is advertised as a highly nutritious breakfast cereal. Product B is a dog biscuit. Unfortunately, this is probably the most accurate commentary on the state of nutrition in the United States that you will ever see. We feed our pets better than we feed ourselves!

How much spinach?

Let's take spinach. I remember as a youngster that Popeye was very popular, and that if I would eat my spinach I could be strong like him. Well, that may have been true in 1948, but it is not true in 1994. Here's why. In 1948 you could buy spinach that had 158 milligrams of iron per hundred grams of spinach. (The current practices of land fertilization were just beginning in 1948.) By 1965 the maximum iron that could be found had dropped to 27 milligrams! In 1973, it was averaging 2.2 mg! That means you would have to eat 75 bowls of spinach today to get the same amount of iron that one bowl might have given you back in 1948![6]

No wonder we all feel low energy and are sickly. We are nutritionally starving to death!

Rice — Another Example

Brown rice is another example. From 1950 to 1975, the protein in brown rice had dropped 10 percent, the calcium 21, percent and the iron, 28 percent.[7]

When you compare brown rice to Minute Rice, you find that the carbohydrates drop from 15 to 7, protein from 154 to 78, calcium from 64 to 5, B2 from .10 to 0, and niacin from 9.4 to 3.3.[8] Processed food is giving you just a fraction of the nutrition that the already depleted natural food would give you. It has been estimated that 65 percent of our foods are processed and 60 percent of us are epidemically sick! Can you suggest one reason why?

Poisoned soil

Not only have we depleted the soil by believing we know better how to crop it than God does, we have poisoned our soil with the use of chemical pesticides which we spray on year after year. Sure, the poisons kill insects. Do you think they might kill or cause cellular mutation within our 70 trillion cells also? Yes, they do! So, if at all possible, check out a food co-op (or even a progressive supermarket) and purchase foods which are grown on soil which has not been sprayed with poisons (organically grown).

The book entitled *Our Food, Our World* by the Earth Save Organization states, "In 1990 we had 100,000 percent more chemicals on our farm products than we did in 1945."

On a flight home from Australia last week, I sat next to a dairy farmer and we began talking about farming and the land. He said that in the last five years they have been putting many more chemicals on the land than ever before. And his son (who is only in his thirties) was just operated on for prostate cancer.

Second Chronicles 7:14 speaks of a way of healing our land, I believe, both spiritually and physically. They always go hand in hand. It says, "If my people, who are called by my name, will humble themselves and pray, and seek My face and **turn from their wicked ways**, then will I hear from heaven, forgive their sin, and heal their land." I wonder if one of the wicked ways we need to turn from is the chemical poisoning of the land.

You may say, "It is hard to eat natural foods, especially since my lifestyle requires me to eat at restaurants quite often." Well, that is why we have a future chapter on antioxidants. Antioxidants will help clean up the free radicals which are produced in your body. Plus, there are some incredibly healthy food products which you can eat which can make up for much of what is lacking in American food products. We will discuss them in just a few minutes.

At the very least you will want to wash the fruits and vegetables which you purchase at the grocery store with a non-toxic natural cleanser. Even bananas should be washed because their skins are covered with extremely toxic chemicals. If you touch the unwashed peel of the banana and then touch the banana, you have effectively carried the poison to the banana and into your stomach.

Dead food

The law in America requires that all processed food be dead before it is placed on the supermarket shelves. (That is why it is best to eat the fresh, unprocessed food found around the circumference of most stores.) Processed food has generally been heated to a sustained temperature in order to kill off bacteria. However, the natural enzymes in food begin to die at 107 degrees, and are completely dead at 120 degrees. So all the processed food is dead food. Now dead food can SUSTAIN life (at a poor level). It just can't NOURISH life and make you feel vitalized! I recommend you take a capsule of live enzymes with your meals if you find your lifestyle forces you to eat a fair amount of processed or cooked foods. I have begun to, and I believe it makes a huge difference. If your body doesn't have the right tools to work with, it is hard for it to keep you healthy and vital.

Stripped food

Our methods of processing foods generally strip away all its natural goodness and leave us with things like white flour (which we then seek to enrich with a few vitamins), or white sugar (which no insect or animal will invade because it can't live on it). Such a system is like being mugged, and then having the mugger come back, after taking your wallet and other personal belongings, and hand you a $10 bill from your wallet, telling you that you are "enriched." I don't think so. This is what has been done with most processed foods. They are stripped of their natural goodness and then enriched with a few vitamins.

For example, with the advent of the steal roller mill in 1890, we discovered how to take wheat and remove the germ, which has all the nutrients in it, and remove the shell, which has all the bran and fiber associated with it, and now make the best donuts on the face of the earth. We have taken out 95 percent of the nutrition that was originally there, and we add back a small portion with piles of worthless sugar which actually tax our bodies to process.

In 1993, the average American ate 160 pounds of white sugar, 95 percent in non-discretionary forms (i.e. foods we purchase which have white sugar in them). For example, "Twinkies" have twelve teaspoons of sugar in each one, and the average can of pop has nine or ten teaspoons of sugar. Research has shown that twenty- four teaspoons of sugar eaten in one day reduces the number of bacteria that our white blood cells will destroy by 92 percent![9] No wonder I always felt that eating sugar when I had a cold allowed the cold to gain ground during the next several hours. It did gain ground, because my immune system was temporarily incapacitated.

Chemical additives

To make sure food has a long shelf-life, we currently add three thousand chemical additives, many of them potent vitamin and mineral blockers. Eighteen thousand of these chemicals had not cleared the FDA's safety procedures as of December 31, 1990 (according to *Our Food, Our World* by the Earth Save Organization).

These chemicals are totally foreign to our bodies and have to be flushed out by the immune system, along with any of our additional cells which the chemicals cause to mutate. Talk about burdening the immune system! We currently live in the most toxic environment in the history of the world and we have the most toxic bodies ever experienced. No wonder the immune system cannot keep up and gets behind, allowing cancer cells and other mutated cells to propagate, producing killer diseases. Our immune system needs some help if we are to live long, healthy lives.

Do you think the FDA, which approves all these chemicals, has done a study on the **cumulative effects all these toxins** have on our bodies when they are all ingested over a week or a month or a lifetime? I would certainly hope they have. Guess what — THEY HAVEN'T! Yet they assure us everything is okay. It is not okay. One in three people have or will get cancer. There must be a reason for it. I had hoped the FDA was looking out for me. I believe they have fallen down in their responsibility. It is time I become responsible for my own health. Those who said they were responsible are doing some very irresponsible things. I want to know what all these chemicals and toxins **taken together** do to my body. Actually, I already know. The death statistics tell me. The Bible says we can judge according to fruit. This fruit is deadly.

Chemical food

And then, of course, we have many products which cannot really be classed as food (even though we eat them). They are synthetic, chemical combinations which will last for 100 years on the shelf and not spoil. You see, **real food** spoils. Chemical and synthetic junk doesn't. Perhaps this is why the Surgeon General of the United States said in 1988 that one half of the Americans who die do so because of what we put in our mouths. I wonder if it is a sin to commit slow suicide by ingesting all this junk and leaving our spouses without a mate and our children as orphans.

Here are two principles which can help you choose what to eat: 1) Eat only foods which spoil — just eat them before they do! 2) Stay away from everything white (white sugar, white flour, fat and salt). These two cautions will put you miles ahead of most other Americans.

One gentlemen I read about has a Twinkie which is almost fifteen years old. He opens it up each year to see how it is doing. It's doing great! Let me give you a hint: If it hasn't spoiled in fifteen years, it isn't food! You might want to put it in the "unclean" category.

A Testimony from the Farm

I grew up on a farm, and I had a great-aunt who lived totally naturally when it came to foods. She was always against farmers who added chemicals to their lands and put "pills" in their sugar trees when they tapped them. We did both. I remember my father remarking about how unfounded her concerns were. However, my father has been operated on for the removal of cancer while in his 60's, while my aunt is now over 100 years of age and is still in good health, with no cancer. Perhaps she was right after all.

My decision on land and food

In the areas of land and food, I believe we have violated the spirit of the laws of Leviticus (which is purity, or, "Don't eat junk!"). My personal decision is to eat, as much as possible, unprocessed natural foods. Then, since I can't totally separate myself from this twentieth century mess, I take vitamins, antioxidants, herbs and enzymes to clean up the rest of the cellular destruction caused by living in modern civilization. I also exercise regularly, try to live in faith, hope and love, and then, ultimately, trust the Lord for healing, health and strength.

You can add a "super-food" which nourishes your cells

Many people are like Patti and me, and really do not have time or interest in developing their own natural garden or joining a food co-op. We are also often on the road and are forced to eat out so much that it would literally be impossible to live on vitalized natural foods. But we have found something we can do. We have discovered that there are "super-foods" which can give to our bodies the nourishment they need — nourishment they are not getting from today's devitalized lands and foods. A super-food is extremely rich in a large variety of vitamins, minerals, trace minerals and amino acids, and very highly assimilable by our bodies.

In my research, I have found two such super-foods (there may be more): 1) blue-green algae, and 2) green barley leaves. My first reaction to both of these was very negative. First, I did not want to eat algae, nor barley leaves. Luckily, I don't have to. Both are available in capsule form. Second, I just felt the claims of both were too far-fetched to be realistic. How could they be THAT important to our diets? Well, if we were eating crops grown on living land, that had not been mined and chemically treated, these two foods would probably not be that important. However, since most of us are not, they become much more important. More about the reasons why later.

To compare these two foods, I tried them both, and researched them both, and became convinced that I prefer the algae. Here are some reasons for my decision: 1) I experienced a "tissue cleansing" while on the algae, which I didn't while on the barley. (Tissue cleansing will be explained later.) 2) Algae is the most basic food of the entire planet. Everything comes from it. 3) Kim Bright Cassano, a nationally recognized nutritionist, had been on barley green for years and has switched to blue-green algae. She told me that algae was like rocket fuel when compared to the barley.

Blue-Green Algae

Medical science has so far identified sixteen "gross" elements and forty-three "trace" elements which are of vital importance to the healthy maintenance of the human system. According to U.S. Senate Document No. 264, 99 percent of Americans are mineral deficient! Eighty elements and trace elements have been identified in blue-green algae (some are in very small amounts, and only twenty-three are listed on the label), as well as twelve vitamins and twenty amino acids.

Blue-green algae is also **97% assimilable** by our bodies, so we get essentially all its goodness. Most foods do not even come close to this level of availability.

When your body has all necessary elements, it is healthy and immune to disease by its very nature. Food is intended to furnish the body with all the live elements needed for the regeneration of its cells and tissues. If the body fails to be healthy, the lack or deficiency of regenerative elements in the food is the cause of, and the responsibility for, whatever ailment, sickness or disease overtakes it. Our bodies seek homeostasis, equilibrium or balance. This equals health.

When given the right building blocks to work with, the body maintains itself in health.

I found it hard to believe that the minute amounts of trace elements listed on a bottle of blue-green algae could ever affect an entire human body. Then I read a statement by Dr. Norman Walker:

"You cannot conceive the very small microscopic amount of each
trace element which the body must have in order to be **VIBRANTLY
HEALTHY**. Some parts and functions of the body need only one or
two trace elements. For example: the sinovial fluid, and lubricating
substance in the joints, require Bismuth. The outer skin of the body
needs Chromium. The appendix needs Erbium. The pineal gland
needs both Iridium and Lithium...."[10]

By taking just a bit of this wonderful food (in capsule form) as a
supplement to your diet, you will find many wonderful things happen
to your body. Essentially, the nourishment will give your body the
needed resources to rebuild any broken or damaged parts and improve
your body's chances of returning to homeostasis. Testimonies of its
power range from improved eyesight, to relief from back pain, to better
scores in sports by world champion competitive athletes. Generally,
one will experience feelings of increased energy and vitality; reduction
and alleviation of stress, anxiety and depression; relief from the discom-
forting symptoms of fatigue, hypoglycemia, some allergies, poor digestion and sluggishness; and improved memory and mental clarity.
People also experience elimination of mood swings, toxin elimination,
better sleep, reduced cravings for food and sweets, lower blood pressure and many other health benefits.

Then there are many specialized health problems which have disappeared as people's bodies receive adequate nutrition through the algae.
Prostate problems have been normalized, as well as triglycerides, arthritis and diabetes, and many other severe and degenerative diseases.
Basically, any and every disease will be fought off by your body, if it has
the right tools to fight with. Algae gives it the right tools.

You just need to **try it** for thirty days and see what it may do for you.
If your body needs detoxifying first, you will experience a bit of a "tissue
cleansing" during the first few days or weeks of taking the algae as your
body cleanses itself. (See the chapter on tissue cleansing.)

I did not anticipate any tissue cleansing when I began taking these
products because I had been eating the Genesis diet for several months,
had just finished fasting with the use of herbs and bentonite to help
cleanse my intestines, was drinking living water, and was taking vitamins and antioxidants. Yet I found several reactions during the first
and second week which I would class as a mini tissue cleansing as my
body detoxified. (Perhaps I have had other cleansings in the past but
have been unaware of them, being ignorant of them and their symptoms.) During the first two days I became very sleepy, and the skin on

my feet cracked and broke. Then I began to simply experience out-standing energy. It was truly exciting to feel such vitality, and I had many more vivid dreams and awakened earlier. I was becoming enthu-siastic about this product which at first had seemed offensive to me.

A Testimony of Blue-Green Algae's Restorative Powers

We received the following testimony from Don Santini:

"My wife, Charlotte, and I are feeling so much better since we became involved with [blue-green algae]. My wife has had rheuma-toid arthritis for over seven years. She took steroids — gold shots — and many other expensive special vitamin supplements, plant from chiropractors, etc., and she has never received any real results that she could live with. When she was on the steroid program instituted by her arthritis doctors, she had bad side effects. She normally weighs 110 - 115 pounds. On the steroid program, she gained so much weight it scared her. She weighed in at 165. That's pretty heavy for a 5'4" lady. We got her off the steroids and on a nutritional food program and she improved some and went back down to 106 - 110 pounds. After a couple of years she started getting worse again and we had reached the point that we had received delivery of her motorized wheelchair. We did this because she became very re-stricted in where we could go because if she had to walk more than 300 - 400 yards, she paid for it with increased pain and increased inflammation in her joints which it then took extra time to begin to feel normal again.

"We heard of the...blue-green algae from Walt Childs and what it had done for him and his wife. We enrolled in [the company], or-dered product and started on a program of vital nutrition, even Super Nutrition, if you will. She had a slight fever, headache and upset stomach the first day and evening. She felt much better the next morning, but when she got out of bed and started moving around, she noticed increased pain in her joints.

"We were really glad we were warned that this might happen, even that it probably would happen. She was prepared to have increased pain in her joints for 4 or 5 days and maybe for an entire month. After about 4 or 5 days, she started feeling much better than she has for seven years. She first noticed she can almost close her hand and the pain is really diminished. Next her knees started feeling better, with the swelling in her knee and back of her knee going down some. Then she started doing something she has not done for seven years. She started getting a full night's sleep. For the past seven years she has always had restless sleep because every time she would move, it would wake her up with the pain.

"She now has more energy than she has had for many years. I recently pinched a nerve in my back and neck and it has basically limited me drastically. I have not been able to mow our lawn (over one acre) and it had really gotten out of control. Last Saturday, against my will, she decided to mow the yard. She worked for over three hours pushing our mower. It has a five horse motor but does not propel the mower at all. She did that all herself. After three hours or more mowing the lawn, she came in the house at 7:30 that evening and decided it was time to clean up the kitchen. Then she baked a peach cobbler and at 9:00 P.M. she finally sat down and relaxed. She did not have adverse reactions to all she had done. This would have been absolutely impossible four weeks ago.

"You just might understand why I am so excited about discovering [blue-green algae]. In four weeks it has changed my wife's and my lives. I haven't had this much energy since I was a teenager and that was over 40 years ago...."

What Makes Blue-Green Algae So Special?

Some algaes which are sold on the market are grown in manmade ponds into which man puts the amounts of chemicals he deems prudent, according to the timing he thinks is prudent. Blue-green algae is different. It is grown in a natural lake along the southern border of Oregon. Volcanic actions in past history have deposited thirty-five feet of mineral-rich volcanic ash and rock at the bottom of this shallow warm lake. This 594,000 acre lake can produce an excess of 200 million pounds of its unique strain of Aphanizomenon flos-aquae annually, which is enough to feed every person on the face of the planet one to two grams each day. The top one-inch of sediment at the bottom of the lake contains enough nutrients to support this massive annual bloom of algae for 60 years — even without any new nutrients coming into the lake! Blue-green algae is freeze-dried right at the lake, in order to preserve its natural properties. We have made blue-green algae a part of our lives.

If You Are a Farmer

If you till the land, the following are some steps which you can take to restore it to life and vitality. Albert Ocker may be contacted for consultation purposes.

1. Add high-calcium lime which separates the soil particles and provides one of the most important ingredients for the growing plant.

2. Stop using anhydrous ammonia — a product which was developed during the Korean War to make soil hard enough to make runways. Farmers put it on to get more nitrogen in their soils.

3. Put biological life back in through proper compost, manures or fish fertilizers.

4. Apply natural phosphorus to the soil to bring it to the proper balance.

5. Run over the land with AerWay equipment which shatters the soil eight inches deep so you get deep penetration of air and water. This will reactivate normal bacteria growth.

Various liquid and dry products have been formulated which can be applied to the land or to crops which will raise the brix within a week. This is a temporary stimulant to get one through a critical situation. However, all the above steps should be done in a normal situation.

If You Grow Your Own Garden

If you grow your own garden, there are several things you can do to increase the nutritional value of your produce. Albert Ocker shared these with me, and is willing to have you call him for additional information.

1. Till and plant oats in fall and by spring you will have ready mulch.

2. Dust plants with feed-grade calcium and dynamacious earth mixed together for insect control.

3. For additional fertilizer, apply directly to top of earth S K Blend plus feed-grade calcium, 50 to 100 pounds of each per acre. (Call Mr. Ocker for ordering information.) This will create an environment for earthworms and bacteria to grow in the soil.

Research has shown that organic food averages a mineral concentration twice that of foods grown on commercially fertilized lands, plus it has four times more nutritional trace elements (such as boron, calcium, iodine, chromium, magnesium and zinc). Finally organic food has lesser toxic trace elements.

The Difference Between Organic and Natural

While organic food is definitely an improvement over chemically grown, it is important to keep two considerations in mind.

1. Organic can be as toxic as chemicals. If the manure from cattle has an imbalance of minerals, it can be very toxic to the land. And, if the manure comes from animals which have been eating crops grown on devitalized and imbalanced land, their manures represent the same devitalization and imbalance.

2. Not all organic things are biologically safe — some can drive out biological activity. Again Albert Ocker is willing to serve as a consultant to you.

Additional Resources on the Soil

Albert I. Ocker, a soil, air and water consultant, is available to both gardeners and farmers. He can offer counsel and equipment for recreating healthy soil. 2181 Roxbury Road, Shippensburg, PA 17257. Phone 717-532-7167.

An outstanding video entitled "Life in the Soil", which discusses in much greater detail what we have covered above, may be ordered from The World Sustainable Agricultural Association, 8554 Melrose Ave., West Hollywood, California 90069.

Acres, U.S.A. Book Store: A Voice for Eco-agriculture, provides a mail order service for many books on the soil. You may get their free catalog by writing P.O. Box 9547, Kansas City, MO 64133. Phone: 816-737-0064. Fax 816-737-3346. Special books of interest in the discussion of the soil include:

An Acres U.S.A. Primer by Charles Walters and C.J. Fenzau

Life & Energy in Agriculture by Arden B. Anderson

Science in Agriculture by Arden B. Andersen

Mainline Farming for Century 21 by Dan Skow, D.V.M. &
   Charles Walters

Green Leaves of Barley by Dr. Mary Ruth Swope — Provides an understanding of the tremendous value of eating green barley leaves.

August Celebration by Linda Grover — The story of blue-green algae, how it is grown and processed, and why it is so valuable to eat. Written as an autobiography, it is a fun and interesting book to read. You will find it enjoyable and refreshing as long as you recognize that it is not written from an evangelical perspective.

You may order a refractometer (cost about $230) from J & J Agri-products & Services Inc, 220 South Second Street, Dillsburg PA 17109. Phone 717-432-2461 or 1-800-233-0138. This mail order company will also send you a catalog of other products they have available for growing healthy natural crops and for testing your land.

References

[1] Gerson, Max, *A Cancer Therapy* (Bonita, CA: The Gerson Institute, 1990), p. 14.

[2] Gerson, pp. 176-181.

[3] Wheeler, Philip A. and Ronald B. Ward, *Non Toxic Farming: A Handbook* (TransNational AGronomy, Ltd, 1989), p. 7.

[4] "Don't let soil compaction squeeze your profits," (Indianapolis, IN: Elanco Products Co.) (pamphlet), p. 3.

[5] Wheeler, p. 55.

[6] Grover, Linda, *August Celebration* (Carson City, NV: Gilbert, Hoover & Clark, 1993), p. 33.

[7] Swope, Mary Ruth, *Green Leaves of Barley* (Melbourne, FL: National Preventive Health Services, 1987), p. 24.

[8] Swope, p. 25.

[9] Swope, p. 26.

[10] Walker, N. W., *The Natural Way to Vibrant Health* (Prescott, AZ: Norwalk Press, 1972), p. 111.

Chapter 5

Living Water

"Over 900,000 people get sick each year in the U.S. — and as many as 900 die — from water borne bacterial disease." Source: USA Today, September 27, 1993.

Continuing our discussion of the application of the principle of purity from the book of Leviticus to our twentieth century living, we will investigate the healing power of pure water.

The water we drink violates the spirit of the law of purity

Today we add chlorine, ammonia, and fluoride to our drinking water, run it through pipes with lead solder on the joints, and drink it, hoping the chlorine has killed all bacteria (and doesn't kill us) and that the fluoride will strengthen our teeth.

Chlorine

Sure enough, chlorine does kill bacteria (single-celled plants). But what do you think it does to the 70 trillion cells within your body? Do you think it just stops killing because it hits your lips, or do you think it goes right on killing off and damaging and mutating these little cells? If you guessed the latter, you are right. One simple way of noting the damage chlorine does to cellular tissue is to notice how bloodshot your eyes become after swimming underwater with them open in a chlorinated swimming pool. The chlorine has killed and damaged many cells in your eyes.

Chlorinated drinking water is directly responsible for more than 4,200 cases of bladder cancer and 6,500 cases of rectal cancer every year (based on a study published in the American Journal of Public Health and conducted by the Medical College of Milwaukee). Chlorine reacts with other substances in water to form chloroform, carbon tetrachloride, toluene, xylene, styrene and other cancer-causing compounds (carcinogens). The only question is whether enough of these carcinogens are produced to cause cancer in your body. Every carcinogen that goes into your body causes some damage which must be fixed up by the immune system. The question is, "When does the build-up from so many sources finally overload the immune system, and mutated cells begin growing faster than the immune system can destroy them?" I personally don't think I want to experiment on my body to find out. I will get the chlorine out of my water with a water treatment unit at my kitchen tap.

In a Montreal study, families who did not filter their own water suffered 51 percent more colds, flu and digestive problems than did those who drank filtered water.

A National Academy of Sciences study in 1975 revealed thousands of organic chemicals in the drinking water of eighty cities. This is because we have polluted our ground water with literally thousands of organic chemicals. The committee determined that volatile organic compounds make up 10 percent by weight of the total organic matter in water.

By the mid-1980's, the EPA (Environmental Protection Agency) had reported that thousands of wells had been closed because of contaminated water. Nitrates and over sixty farm pesticides had been identified.

The EPA Environmental News on May 11, 1993 reported, "In 819 water systems across the country, lead levels were above the EPA 'action level' of 15 parts per billion."

So what do you do? You could go to the store and buy bottled water. However, since the FDA's chemical contamination standards for bottled water are the same as the EPA's standard for tap water, you never know what you are getting when you buy bottled water. The contaminants which can be in your tap water can legally be in bottled water sold in stores. A study done in California last year showed that about 25% of the bottled water sold in California was simply tap water sold as bottled water.

One possible solution is to put a good water purifier at the tap in your kitchen sink. Because hot steaming water with chlorine gas escaping from it cannot be healthy to breathe while you shower, you probably want one at your shower also. One alarming study in the American

Journal of Public Health, July 1992, suggested that two-thirds of the harmful effects of chlorine are due to inhalation and skin absorption from showering in chlorinated water. Remember, every bit you can do to detoxify your body helps.

It is a bit of a chore to find a good water treatment unit. You can use granulated activated carbon, which is great for removing pesticides and other contaminants. It "holds" these in its structure thereby "cleaning up" the water. The negative side is that activated carbon is an excellent environment for bacterial contamination. In addition, it not only can grab and hold on to contaminants, but it can also release those contaminants unexpectedly. This can happen when the water changes temperature or pH rather quickly. Drinking water from a filter which is releasing its "hold" means you are drinking water many times worse than with no filter at all! This can be solved by back flushing one's system at 140 degrees.

There are water distilling units available which take everything out of the water, including all minerals. However, your body needs minerals, so this may not be the best course of action either.

What about reverse osmosis? It is much more expensive. It does take all minerals out of the water, so you need additional supplementation in order to restore the minerals which have been removed. The other problem is that it takes three gallons of water to get one gallon back. However, on the bright side, it does get rid of ALL bacteria.

Living Water

We do have a simple solution for the bacteria and carcinogens that are in our water supply. It was given by God to an Austrian naturalist and inventor, Johann Grander. He has developed what he calls the "Living Water System." It is a water treatment system which is put on the incoming line to your home, farm, factory, hospital, etc. This amazing invention turns dead water into living water and does the following:

- It oxygenates water, increasing the aerobic bacteria functioning.
- The increased aerobic bacteria reduce pathenogetic bacteria **without the use of chemicals**.
- It removes about 80 percent of the odors from water.
- It changes the charge of water from a negative ion charge to a positive ion charge, thus putting the toxins in your body (which normally have a negative charge) into suspension and flushing them out of your system.

- It is beneficial for livestock, pets and aquariums.
- It restores lakes and rivers back to health.
- It provides healthier plant growth (20 to 40 percent improvement).
- It reduces odors caused by bacteria and enhances cleaning.

Sometime in 1994, the New England Journal of Medicine will be publishing the results of a major study on this Living Water System, discussing its health benefits. Over 50,000 Living Water units have been sold in Europe, Austria and Australia in the last 12 years. This invention is just now coming to the United States and Canada in 1994.

What Makes the Living Water System Work?

You probably know that a fresh flowing mountain stream will cleanse itself of harmful pollutants within a few miles of flowing downstream. God has created it this way. I never thought much about why this was. I just accepted it as fact. Of course, in an industrialized nation, it may not be so, because of the acid rain, and constant flow of pollutants into the stream. Streams may no longer be able to do what they were designed to do.

Johann Grander feels that God has shown him that the water in its natural state is energized by three types of magnetic energies. It has been proven through homeopathy that water has a remarkable memory and capacity to store energy. With this in mind, Johann Grander has discovered a way to re-introduce these three vital magnetic energies into water. The result is that we can have "living water" in our homes, offices and swimming pools any time we want.

What happens when water runs over gravel and stones? The volcanic process by which these stones were produced causes them, over time, to align their electromagnetic energies in accordance with the North and South poles of earth's polarity. The water in turn structures itself according to this global electromagnetic field. The molecules realign themselves and coalesce into large families, regenerating themselves. Therein comes the extensive cleansing power of water. Johann Grander's procedure is successful because it duplicates the efficient process of nature.

Prof. Gerhard Pioch has found that the residues of poisonous water contaminants have a harmful negative polarity. In this state it is difficult for the body to eliminate these compounds. The Living Water System reverses this by changing the polarity from negative to positive. Only then is your body able to cleanse itself. About 70 percent of your body weight is water. The re-introduction of water with a positive ion charge into your body can stimulate tremendous health effects.

In a long-term study, two middle-aged people (a man and a woman) were asked to daily drink two liters of Living Water and to bathe in Living Water. An examination of their bathing water and their urine showed 50(!) different, mostly chemical, waste matters that had reached their bodies by way of food, medications or in a similar manner. Among those were chemicals that have been prohibited for several years, traces of E 605, DDT, poisonous heavy metals, etc. The regular drinking of Living Water and bathing reduced the residues of the poisonous and waste matters and enabled their precipitation within five or six weeks.

Through the technique of implosion, the Living Water System re-imprints natural magnetic vibrations on our drinking water, in much the same way that sound is recorded on a blank audio tape. The Living Water System contains highly energized water that imparts information and energy to our drinking water as it passes through it. During this process the amount of dissolved oxygen in the water is also increased.

The following is an interesting picture of a drop of normal tap water and a drop of Johann Grander's Living Water. The pictures were taken by Kirlian photography, and show the enhanced life force present in the living water. [1]

Many people have seen remarkable health results after installing a Living Water Unit and beginning to drink and bathe in Living Water. Under scientific research in Europe, it was found that toxins appeared in both the bathing water and the urine of those drinking and bathing

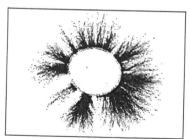

Normal Tap Water

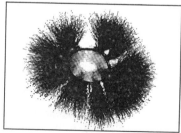

Grander *"Living Water"*

The energy field of water as displayed by Kirlian Photography.
Water drops show the difference between tap water and energized, "Living Water.

in Living Water. And some of the toxins which appeared had been off the market for many years, such as DDT.

Following are some results we have seen through the use of the Living Water System. One friend of ours put a unit on his swimming pool and the algae in his pool cleared up without chemicals. (In order to keep the pool clear, sea salt needed to be added). Solid deposits in septic systems disappear after just two weeks, and the water in these septic tanks become crystal clear a while later. Patti noticed that her vases that held her flowers no longer developed a film on the inside. We noticed that the swirl in the water going down our sink drain was reversed after going through the Living Water unit, giving us conclusive visual proof that something indeed had changed in the water.

The unit does the entire house, never wears out, has no replaceable parts and uses no electricity. So it is a once-in-a-lifetime investment for good health, and as such, is probably one of the better investments you will make. It can be purchased with monthly payments.

A Clear Brook Unit for Your Kitchen Faucet

The Living Water System mentioned above does not actually filter anything out of the water. The only claim they have made at the time of writing this book was, "What seems to happen...is that the living water system transports these chemicals, toxins, heavy metals, and so on, right through the human system without doing any damage." The phrase "seems to happen" does not convince me of anything, so I decided that I wanted to drink water that had passed through a filter to get some of the chemicals out. I researched a bit to see if I could discover an effective and inexpensive unit which would sit next to the kitchen faucet for drinking and cooking water.

Both distillation units and reverse osmosis units take almost all the minerals out of the water, and my body needs minerals. Some have said that the minerals in water cannot be absorbed by our bodies anyway. We must get them through the foods we eat. Others maintain that the minerals found in water can be partially used by our bodies. I have not been able to discover the truth on this issue.

Both distillation units and reverse osmosis are quite expensive to purchase and to maintain. An inexpensive distillation unit costs about $400. With reverse osmosis, it takes six hours of processing to get one or two gallons of water through the unit.

I personally settled on a Clear Brook unit. It is tested and guaranteed to last for 10,000 gallons of water (or five years) before you need to replace the filter. That is several times longer than many other units on the market. The unit does not build up bacteria within it because of silver in its inner construction. (Silver inhibits bacterial growth.) It removes chlorine, chemicals and pesticides, and the counter top unit only costs $132. So the cost of purifying your drinking and cooking water is down to $.01 or $.02 per gallon. Only three water filter units are approved for sale in California. This is one of them.

New water purification units are appearing on the market all the time, making fantastic claims. Be careful! If you cannot personally verify the claims through your own knowledge, find someone who can. I have called my brother-in-law, who is a high school science teacher, several times to check on the validity of my research. He has helped me find several false claims in advertising.

Water heals

Dr. F. Batmanghelidj, M.D. has written an entire book on water, entitled, *Your Body's Many Cries For Water*. He has published an account of his own clinical observations as he successfully treated more than 3000 peptic ulcer sufferers with water alone. This report was published as the editorial article in the "Journal of Clinical Gastroenterology" in June of 1983. He has found that less severe cases of peptic ulcer sufferers achieve total pain relief in about eight minutes.

He feels that the last signal of your body's dehydration is a "dry mouth." By then much damage has already been done to your body. The July 1994 issue of "Consumer Reports on Health" confirm his belief, quoting the following study.

"The University of Nevada researchers recruited 13 men over age 60 to hike through the desert for two hours without a drop to drink. By weighing the men before and after that ordeal, the researchers were able to calculate how much fluid each man had sweated away. Later, the men returned to the desert for another two-hour trek. This time, the researchers provided bottles containing the amount of water each man would be expected to lose through sweating, and they encouraged the men to drink along the way. But the men still drank less than two-thirds as much fluid as they lost.

"Put to the same test, six men under age 35 did drink enough to offset their fluid loss, confirming earlier research showing that younger exercisers do get thirsty enough in the heat. But older people apparently do not get as thirsty. Therefore, they should try to drink about half again as much as it takes to quench their thirst."[2]

Dr. F. Batmanghelidj is also convinced that early morning sickness of a pregnant mother is a thirst signal of both the fetus and the mother.

Scientific research shows that water is a solvent and means of transport within your body. It also has an essential hydrolytic role in all aspects of body metabolism — water dependent chemical reactions (hydrolysis). At the cell membrane, the osmotic flow of water can generate "hydroelectric" energy that is stored in the energy pools. Thus water, the solvent of the body, regulates all functions, including the activity of the solutes it dissolves and circulates.

Dr. Batmanghelidj says that the major types of pain which your body will utilize to tell you that it is in a drought condition are: dyspepsia (heart burn), rheumatoid arthritis pain, anginal pain (heart pain on walking), low back pain, headaches and leg pain on walking. Anyone suffering any of these pains would be wise to try water therapy for 30 days and just see if six or eight glasses of water a day would take care of them. Wouldn't that be an easy and inexpensive way to get healed? It sure can't hurt anything to try it! (Incidentally, Dr. Batmanghelidj has an interesting section on what causes AIDS and how to cure it in his book on water. He suggests that there is no HIV virus but there is another cause altogether. I have heard similar confirming discussion along these lines.)

Healed by a three-day water fast

Dr. Norman Walker speaks of the healing power of water in one of his books. He was taught and personally confirmed in his own life's experience that if one is sick, he can go on a three-day water fast, simply drinking a glass of water every hour, and after three days he will be well. Hey, it's worth a try! Sounds like a low-cost experiment to me, with few toxic side effects. If it worked, it would sure be worth it. If it didn't, you would still have saved some money on food, cleansed your body of toxins, and enhanced your prayer life. Sounds to me like you win either way. That makes it a very low-risk experiment.

How much water should you drink a day?

Take your body weight, divide by two and drink that many ounces of water per day. So if you weigh 170 pounds, you would drink 85 ounces of water per day or about seven 12 oz. glasses. Dr. Batmanghelidj states that the absolute minimum amount of water you should take in during a day is six to eight 8-ounce glasses.

Should one drink water with meals?

I have heard for years that it is healthier not to drink water with your meals because it dilutes the digestive enzymes in your stomach. However, I have still done it because I feel thirsty when I eat, and I do like to honor the call which my body itself is making upon me. I believe that hearing what life itself is saying is an important consideration in knowing truth.

I was excited to see two specialists agree with what my body was telling me. One is Dr. F. Batmanghelidj, M.D. As an expert in your body's use of water, he says you should drink water at meal time. "Adjusting water intake to meal-times prevents the blood from becoming concentrated as a result of food intake. When the blood becomes concentrated, it draws water from the cells around it."[3]

A second expert on water and digestive enzymes is Jeffrey Bland Ph.D., who wrote the booklet "Digestive Enzymes", part of the series entitled "A Good Health Guide" and edited by Dr. Richard A. Passwater. In his book, he, too, says that in order for your digestive enzymes to work properly you need a couple of glasses of water with your meal. "It is known that the heaviest secretion of enzymes from the pancreas occurs one to two hours after a meal and that fluids taken with the meal stimulate gastric secretion for optimal acidity in the stomach and promote enzyme and bicarbonate secretion in the small intestine. This contradicts the seemingly logical notion many people have, that fluids with the meal dilute the enzymes and prevent proper digestion, but the evidence seems quite clear that sufficient fluid with the meal is essential for stimulating gastric, pancreatic and intestinal responses. The liquid should be preferably at room temperature, in the amount of one or two glasses, for optimal intestinal function."[4]

I appreciated these experts' confirming witness to the message that my body was telling me. I find it is quite easy to drink a couple of glasses of water with each meal, and thus simply fulfill my body's requirement for six to eight glasses of water per day.

One piece of information that did adjust me a bit. You may have noticed that Dr. Bland recommended that you not drink ice cold water with your meal as that slows or halts the digestive process. It is much better to drink warmer water with your meals. It is also helpful to put a piece of lemon in your water as it aids the liver's functions. These changes I can easily make. I'll save the ice cold water for the middle of the afternoon and early morning when I awaken.

It is wise to avoid beer, caffeine, sugar and chemicals in your drinks as these must all be filtered out through the 30 billion filtering cells in one's kidneys. Excessive amounts of these products end up causing damage to one's body.

Even processed juices may have chemical preservatives added and will have lost most of their original nutritional value. On the other hand, freshly squeezed juices drunk within an hour of being squeezed are incredibly detoxifying and nourishing to your body, and should be taken as much as possible. Both Dr. Gerson and Dr. Walker recommend them highly. Dr. Walker says rather than drink six or eight glasses of water in a day, he will drink six or eight glasses of freshly squeezed fruit and vegetable juices. He only drinks one glass of water upon awakening.

Dr. Gerson at the Gerson Institute puts his patients on 13 or more glasses of freshly squeezed fruit and vegetable juices per day and finds that it detoxifies the body so fast that cancerous tumors disappear. The doctors at the Gerson Institute are experts at healing cancer through nutrition and have been doing it for about 50 years. Dr. Gerson also has his patients taking enemas every four hours because so many toxins are being released to the liver that if it is not continuously cleansed, the toxins will build up in the liver and cause death. This, unfortunately, happened with some of his early patients, before he discovered the need for enemas. So anyone seeking to follow Dr. Gerson's approach would first want to purchase his books which describe his process in detail, to be sure of following every step of it. Or one may want, instead, to become a patient at the Gerson Institute for three or four weeks, so you are under expert medical supervision. I would suggest the latter.

What a wonderful age of discovery we live in! I pray we make the most of it and heal our bodies as well as our environment.

Additional Resources

Living Water by Viktor Schauberger available through Acres U.S.A. bookstore.

Your Body's Many Cries for Water by F. Batmanghelidj, M.D.

Become Younger by Dr. N.W. Walker, D. Sc. If you read Dr. Walker, you will note that he promotes primarily raw fruits and vegetables, and doesn't even like starches (which are in the Genesis diet). May I suggest that the healing part of the Genesis diet is the fruits and vegetables, the filler part is the starches.

References

[1] Grander Living Water (Vancouver, BC: Ecolife Technology) pamphlet

[2] "Fitness Update," Consumer Reports on Health, volume 6, number 7 (July 1994), 79.

[3] Batmanghelidj, F. *Your Body's Many Cries For Water*, (Falls Church, VA: Global Health Solutions, 1992). pp. 123,124.

[4] Malagelada, J.R. and Go, V.L.W. 1979. Different gastric pancreatic and biliary responses to solid-liquid or homogenized meals. "Digestive Disease Science 24,101," as cited by Bland, Jeffrey, *Digestive Enzymes*, A Good Health Guide Series (New Canaan, CT: Keats Publishing, 1987). p. 9.

Chapter 6

Pure Air and Non-toxic Household Chemicals

The air we breath violates the spirit of the law of purity

The closer you live to the city, the more your air is contaminated. Most of us know that smoke-polluted air causes cancer. So do smog and exhaust, and many other things dumped into our atmosphere. Many things in our homes also produce toxins, including new carpets, new furniture, wall paneling, and the normal household cleaners we depend on every day.

You may want to check a *Consumer Reports* book in your local library to discover a good air purifier for your home so you can reduce this load of toxins you breathe in. It is wise to check various models so that you get what you are paying for. Some have been proven to be valueless.

If you live away from the city, one great way to keep the air more pure in your home is to simply open the window. According to a 1989 report on indoor air quality, submitted to Congress by the Environmental Protection Agency, the nation's worst pollution is found inside our home. Hazardous and toxic chemical concentrations, two to five times higher than outdoors, are found in the typical American home, regardless of whether it is located in rural or industrial areas. In one five-year study, the EPA reported that a number of homes had chemical levels that were 70 times higher inside the home than outside!

So, by simply opening the window in your home, you are provided with one of the cheapest air purifiers you could have.

Some things to look for in a good air purifier

If you decide you want an air purifier, I suggest you get one with a HEPA (High Efficiency Particulate Arresting) filter. These filters were developed by the U.S. Atomic Energy Commission to filter out dangerous radioactive particles, and will take out 99.97 percent of irritating particles (anything larger than .3 microns). The best unit I was able to discover in my research was an Austin HealthMate. Not only does it have a HEPA filter in it, it also has a prefilter of 13 pounds of solid activated carbon and natural zeolite. This removes gases, chemicals, odors, toxins, and vapors (such as secondhand smoke). Its filter uses 80 square feet of pure HEPA media, so it lasts five years without changing. (Some units require their filters to be changed every three to six months). It comes with a five-year warranty and a 60-day money back guarantee. Its cost is $395, and costs an average of $2.55 per month to operate. (That is much cheaper than others I researched.)

Toxic chemicals in our homes violate the spirit of the law of purity

Let's look at another area of toxicity and potential cellular damage which you may have never thought about. You know, it is a wonder any of us are alive, considering all we put our immune systems through in the twentieth century. And the truth is, many of us aren't alive. And those who remain are sickly, have low energy, and often barely feel like living. Hardly the abundant life we were promised when we came to Jesus! However, come to think of it, it was offered to those who kept His commandments. Perhaps by purifying our environments and obeying Biblical laws and principles, we will come alive again. I have, and my prayer is that you will, too!

One booklet which startled me recently was entitled, "Why Are You Poisoning Your Family?" It was filled with statistics concerning the toxicity of the hundreds of chemicals which we use all through our homes every day, and the damaging affects they have on our bodies. Most of these chemicals (i.e. laundry detergents, dishwasher soaps, etc.), are so toxic that if your child were to accidentally drink them, he would have to be rushed to the hospital in hopes that he would live. Now, what do you suppose putting these toxic chemicals on every surface of our homes every day does to our health? Do you think it improves it, or does it give your immune system one more set of problems to fight off? May I suggest the latter? A scientific paper presented by a Vancouver consulting firm at the Indoor Air '90 conference in Toronto, reported that, because of household cleaners, housewives have a 55 percent higher risk of getting cancer than do women working outside the home.

The EPA has reported that toxic chemicals found in every home (from cleaning products to personal care products) are three times more likely to cause cancer than airborne pollutants. More than fourteen years ago, in a 1980 report to the President, the Toxic Substances Strategy Committee stated that the majority of cancers (80 to 90 percent) are triggered by exposure to hazardous substances in the environment. Nervous disorders and respiratory problems are also directly related to environmental pollution.[1]

Seventy thousand new chemicals have been introduced since World War II as by-products of our extensive research into chemical warfare! That's 250 billion pounds of synthetic chemicals produced each year in the United States. According to the U.S. National Research Council, no information on toxic effects is available for 79 percent of the more than 48,500 synthetic chemicals listed by the U.S. Environmental Protection Agency (EPA). Fewer than one-fifth have been tested for acute effects, and fewer than one-tenth, for chronic, reproductive or mutagenic effects.[2]

We Have Been Experimented On!

So WE are the experimental generation! The increase of toxic chemicals on the land, in our homes, in our air, and in our food has all happened since the end of World War II. The extraordinary use of chemicals in every aspect of life, which most of us consider normal, began around 1948. We are the first generation to grow up with such extremely high levels of toxic chemicals in our homes and in our environments. How are we doing in this chemical experiment? How are you doing? How do you feel? Vital, full of life, able to withstand viruses without them making you sick? How are the statistics coming on degenerative diseases and cancer? Are we whipping them, or are they whipping us? Perhaps it is time to bail out of this experiment with a chemicalized world. Perhaps chemicals are not improving our world at all. Perhaps God's world was better before mankind began to "improve" on it. Perhaps it is time the people stand up and say:

"Enough is enough! Don't experiment with poisons in my world any more. If you want to go the moon and experiment with toxic chemicals and see how many a person can ingest before he dies, fine. Just don't do in in my nation and my world any more. This experiment is costing me and my loved ones our lives. And we are dying with horrific pain and suffering, and spending ten or twenty years in horrendous health before we die. I have had enough!"

If you are ready to say this, then you can join with millions of others who have already seen the light and begun saying this years ago. I am joining my voice to this vast multitude as of the writing of this book. I have finally seen the light, and I will do everything I can to put a stop to what I now consider madness, as big business pushes to pollute the world God has given us. If enough of us stop buying, Big Business will stop selling!

A report by the Consumer Product Safety Commission on chemicals commonly found in homes identified 150 chemicals which had been linked to allergies, birth defects, cancer, and psychological abnormalities.

Young children are especially susceptible to these toxins since their higher respiratory rates cause them to inhale three times the amount of contaminants as adults. Plus, they play on the floor which exposes them to asbestos, formaldehyde, and toxic household cleaners.

We know that if you put a chemical against your skin, the chemical will be absorbed through the skin and into the bloodstream. That is why "patches" work for those who are trying to quit smoking. The chemicals in the patch (which is generally attached to the skin on the upper arm) absorb into the bloodstream.

The typical mother washes her children's clothes in a detergent that is so toxic, if you drank it, you could die. Then, she lovingly tucks her babies in at night, dressed in pajamas and covered with bedsheets coated with a residue of toxic detergents. And she does this in the most non-suspecting way, assuming if it is on the grocery store shelf it must be safe. Every surface is cleaned with additional toxic chemicals, and some, such as bathroom tile cleaners and oven cleaners, have fumes so toxic one's breathing is affected for several hours afterward. The detergent used on our dishes could kill us if we drank it, and yet we eat off them, assuming if we can't see any chemical residue with our naked eye, it probably won't hurt us.

Meanwhile, our immune systems work overtime, faithfully detoxifying our bodies day by day, but wishing we would slow down the number of deadly mutants we absorb. Perhaps it is time to give it a break and stop poisoning every surface in our homes and, indeed, many surfaces of our skin, since many toxic chemicals are applied directly to one's skin on a daily basis in the forms of creams and lotions.

Because of testimony by cosmetologists, who claimed that their health problems such as headaches, loss of balance, memory loss, asthma, and irreparable nervous system and respiratory problems, were a result of working with cosmetics, a House subcommittee asked the National Institute of Occupational Safety and Health to analyze 2,983 chemicals used in cosmetics.

"The results were as follows: 884 of the ingredients were found to be toxic. Of these, 314 can cause biological mutation, 218 can cause reproductive complications, 778 can cause acute toxicity, 146 can cause tumors and 376 can cause skin and eye irritation."[3] Wow! Do we really want to play chemist with our skin every morning and put a bunch of these toxic chemicals on our faces? I think not! Even some mouthwashes contain warnings not to swallow them because they contain formaldehyde, ammonia and hydrogen peroxide. Whoa! It is time for a change!

Every year, 5 to 10 million household poisonings are reported. Many are fatal, and most of the victims are children who accidentally ingest common household cleaners. Every day, Americans pour more than 32 million pounds of household cleaning products down the drain, polluting the ground water.

Kare Possick shares the following story in her booklet, *Why Are You Poisoning your Family?* "A friend of mine, named Linda, had sinus problems most of her life. Night time was a particularly miserable time for her, as she couldn't breathe and had to prop herself up on pillows and use nasal sprays and inhalers. Her doctor told her the problem was a deviated septum — so she had it fixed. She had surgery on her nose. Do you know what happened? You probably guessed it — there was absolutely no difference! Yet, Linda now sleeps comfortably and with no congestion. All she changed was her laundry detergent. She changed from the toxic grocery store brands to one that was environmentally sensitive. It made all the difference in the world for her. Interestingly enough, her children's' allergies improved, too!"[4]

I Switched to Non-toxic Products

In my home, we have thrown out all these toxic chemicals, and changed to a wonderful line of household, medicinal, and personal skin-care products made with melaleuca oil (Australian Tea Tree Oil), a natural antiseptic and natural fungicide. This is God's natural medicine rather than man's caustic, synthetic, poisonous compound. It is so natural that you can drink the dish washing detergent without harmful affect. (However, I don't recommend it!)

These wonderful melaleuca products also serve as extremely powerful, and yet very non-toxic, medicines. In the 1920's, Dr. Arthur Penfold found that melaleuca oil was twelve times stronger than carbolic acid (phenol), while being much less toxic to human tissue. It also exhibited unusually potent antifungal activity, more so than any other antiseptic used at that time. It is three to five times more potent than most household disinfectants, and yet totally safe. It has passed the Kelsey-Sykes and the Australian Therapeutic Goods Act tests, the most rigorous antiseptic tests known. A one-in-forty dilution kills antibiotic resistant staph, which are notoriously hard to kill. It can cause complete inhibition of growth, in test tubes, of fungi for up to one month. I have seen it heal athlete's foot in three days, which had resisted doctor's prescribed medicine for years.

Melaleuca oil, a wonderful, God-given, completely natural, non-caustic cleansing and healing agent, has been shown to kill some twenty-three viruses, parasites and bacteria, including staph and strep. It has been used medicinally to cure some thirty-one ailments, including athlete's foot, acne, canker sores, ear infections, genital herpes, and gingivitis, to name a few. We are thrilled that we have been able to replace our caustic household cleansers with this line of household cleansers, personal hygiene items, and medicinal items which contain melaleuca oil. You can make this change also.

In Summary

Rev. Malcolm Smith tells a story about a frustration he faced in the healing ministry. People he prayed for, whom he saw healed of very real diseases, would become sick again with the very same diseases within six months. This troubled him for a great while until one day, while traveling through Belfast, Ireland, he stopped at a juice bar. The owner would crush the juice in front of your eyes, and you could drink some of the healthiest juice in the world. The owner of the juice bar was a raving fanatic for the cause of nutrition. He was the kind of person who swam the Irish Sea, and walked from one end of Ireland to the other sharing his belief that you could live on nuts, grains, berries.

So Malcolm asked him a question. "If all the junk were removed from one's system and a person were healed, and he went back to eating and living the way he had been, how long would it take to get sick again?" The answer he got was, "Here in Northern Ireland, it would take about six months." Wow! After God cleans us out with a divine healing touch, we go right back and pollute our bodies, making ourselves sick again by what we eat and the way we live. He who has ears, let him hear what the Spirit of God is saying to the churches.

I suggest each of us do our best to honor the spirit of the laws of Leviticus, which is to be as pure and clean as possible, and to avoid the unclean. Seek out clean air, clean water, clean food, clean land, and clean household and personal care products. It will do nothing but improve your health by taking a load off your lymphatic system. And you will be bringing health to your entire family. That must be worth something! I do not think I can trust the FDA or the pharmaceutical, fertilizer or chemical companies to keep me safe. There is too much greed and corruption involved. It is time each of us becomes educated about how to take care of our own health. Otherwise, we will join the statistics of those who have traveled the road of degenerative diseases and early death. **This need not be!**

Recommended Reading

Why Are You Poisoning Your Family? by Kare Possick. A small booklet discussing the use of toxic chemicals within the home. Designed to motivate you to make a decision to change to a non- toxic assortment of household products.

Killed on Contact by Cass Igram. One hundred pages showing the healing power of melaleuca oil (tea tree oil), God's finest medicine. It shows its antiseptic qualities, medical uses, uses with fungal diseases, uses as an insecticide and personal-hygiene uses.

References

[1] Dadd, Debra Lynn, *Non-Toxic, Natural and Earthwise* (Jeremy P. Tarcher, 1990), as cited by Possick, Kare, *Why Are You Poisoning Your Family?* (Madeira Beach, FL: Kare Possick, 1994), p. 4.

[2] Dadd, as cited by Possick, p. 3.

[3] Sokol, Nancy Green, *Poisoning Our Children* (Noble Press, 1991) as cited by Possick, p. 29.

[4] Possick, p. 23.

Chapter 7

Detoxifying the Body Through Proper Bowel Management

As we have learned in earlier chapters, the three foundational rules for good health are to: 1) build your immune system, 2) detoxify your body, and 3) nourish your cells. This chapter deals with effectively detoxifying your body through having a healthy elimination system.

When I first discovered colon cleansing, I found it a bit disgusting and decided I would not deal with it at all, or if I did, I would put the information in a single paragraph. However, when I read Bernard Jensen's book entitled *Tissue Cleansing Through Bowel Management*, I was struck by the revelation and insight and healing power of the book, and I began to experiment with enhancing my elimination system. The healing power of proper bowel management is too awesome to skip or to put into a paragraph, so here is a chapter on this amazing way of detoxifying your body.

If your immune system is strong, it will constantly wash all damaged, mutated cells and toxic poisons out of your system. The three ways these damaged cells are discharged are through: 1) the lungs, 2) the bowel and kidneys, and 3) the skin (two pounds per day through the skin). The bowel is supposed to discharge a meal within eighteen hours after it is eaten. In America, because of the type of diet we eat, many people have ten extra meals jammed up in their intestines. If the bowel is stopped up, or only partially functioning, these toxins are not eliminated effectively from your system. Instead they re-circulate and are dumped in areas which create abscesses, open sores, arthritis, headaches, and just about every sickness imaginable. Simply by improving the operation of one's bowel, these built up toxins will be eliminated and the accompanying infirmities can and will be removed. I found this hard to believe at first. A few testimonies and studies helped convince me.

Gerona Alderin tells that as a result of a good colon cleanse, she got rid of lumps on her breasts, restored the color of her eyes to blue, restored great skin color and tone, and abundant energy.[1]

One female patient with rheumatoid arthritis, tells, "When I began the tissue cleansing program, I could hardly use my hands. My left knee was so swollen I couldn't move it. During the program, my hands became more flexible, and the swelling and soreness in the palm of my right hand improved. The swelling in my knee decreased until I could walk without pain. My back is not aching all the time now and seems stronger. My feet aren't so tender on the bottoms."[2]

One patient had open, running ulcers on his feet and was not able to wear socks or shoes. By day seven of the colon cleanse, the open ulcers were healed up! You see, if the toxic poisons can not be eliminated through the colon, they will seek elimination elsewhere. Full color pictures of this amazing seven day healing of the ulcerated feet can be found on page 142 of Bernard Jensen's book.

One study of 1,481 non-nursing women showed that those who are severely constipated tend to have abnormal cells in the fluid extracted from their breasts. Such cells have been found in women with breast cancer and, the researchers suggested, may indicate that the women face an increased risk of developing cancer. The cellular abnormalities occurred five times as often in women who moved their bowels fewer than three times a week, than in women who did so more than once a day. Chronic constipation is often the result of a diet high in protein, fat and refined carbohydrates (sugars and refined flour), but low in such fibrous foods as whole grains, fruits and vegetables.[3] Once again we see that the Genesis diet heals and the American diet kills.

Today there are more than 45,000 laxative and cathartic remedies manufactured and used by Americans alone. It makes you think we might have a problem! Over 70 million Americans suffer from bowel problems. In 1980, over $350 million was spent on laxatives. The number two cause of death in the United States is cancer. Of these, 100,000 give up their lives every year due to cancer of the colon. The American Cancer Society says that evidence in recent years suggests that most bowel cancer is caused by environmental agents. Some scientists believe that a diet high in beef and/or low in fiber is the cause.

Both British and South African medical scientists have studies indicating that people living under primitive conditions on diets high in indigestible fiber passed from 2 1/2 to 4 1/2 times as much feces as those in the Western countries, and these people were found to be relatively free of most of the diseases studied.[4]

Colostomy is a surgical procedure in which the intestine is severed from the colon because of that organ's functional breakdown. The colostomized individual then faces a lifetime elimination of feces through an opening in his side into an attached pouch. There are 100,000 people who undergo this radical approach each year. Proper colon care will prevent this entirely.

Dr. Sir Arbuthnut Lane, who was a surgeon for the King of England, also did colonic surgery and noticed that after surgery many totally "unrelated" diseases were healed in his patients. One young boy, who had arthritis for many years, was in a wheelchair at the time of the surgery. Six months later, this boy had recovered entirely from the disease. Another of his female patients had a goiter which went into remission for the six months following colonic surgery.

These kinds of experiences caused him to see the relationship between a toxic bowel and the functioning of the various organs in the body, and led him to spend the last twenty-five years of his life teaching people how to care for the bowel through nutrition and not surgery. He stated, "All maladies are due to the lack of certain food principles, such as mineral salts or vitamins, or to the absence of the normal defenses of the body, such as the natural protective flora. When this occurs, toxic bacteria invade the lower alimentary canal, and the poisons thus generated, pollute the bloodstream and gradually deteriorate and destroy every tissue, gland and organ of the body."[5]

Dr. John Harvey Kellogg maintained that 90 percent of the diseases of civilization are due to improper functioning of the colon. What this boils down to is that diseased people have toxic bodies, and if they would detoxify their bodies, their diseases would go away.

Of 300 autopsies performed by the National College in Chicago, 285 were found to be constipated. Some were found with bowels nine to twelve inches across and only room for a pencil to pass through, the rest being compacted with encrusted fecal matter. Doctors appear to have the worst death record of any when it comes to intestinal disease. According to the statistics published by the Register General of England, physicians and surgeons ranked at the top of the list, and agricultural laborers at the bottom.

When the bowel fails, the whole body goes into a nutritional crisis. Metabolic shock waves flow to every cell and tissue.

The intestine is to be filled with friendly flora, called acidophilus, producing an acid bowel environment. Bacillus coli is an unfriendly bacteria which grows in an alkaline environment. It is easily produced by having protein for breakfast, lunch, and dinner, or by taking antibiotic drugs. This unfriendly bacteria reach as high as 85 percent of the floral life in the colon of the average American. To restore the proper flora content in one's intestines, one must eat the Genesis diet (i.e. low-fat, low-cholesterol, and high-fiber), and should probably supplement his diet with acidophilus for two to four weeks. You can tell when the flora is changed because your stools are soft, frequent (three times a day), and free from putrid or rancid odor.

Dr. Bernard Jenson has developed a seven-day colon cleanse and has seen triglyceride readings drop from 938 mg/dl (normal is 150 - 200) to 258 mg/dl in one week. At the same time, he has seen cholesterol drop from 348 mg/dl to 277 mg/dl in only seven days.[6] I would have never believed such a thing were possible. But it is surely reasonable if you think about it. Unplug the sewer and the whole backed-up system can be easily cleaned out.

Dr. Jenson believes his seven-day colon cleanse system is the ultimate tissue cleansing system. From my limited studies, I would agree, and if I were severely sick and infected, I would most likely complete it in a flash. It is described in detail in his book *Tissue Cleansing Through Bowel Management*. I personally think everyone should read this book as part of his health education. It is worth its weight in gold. You can do the cleanse at home yourself, which makes it preferable for most people. The alternative is to have a colonic, which is like an advanced enema performed upon you by another person. Most people's modesty would not permit them to go for a colonic. Dr. Jenson recommends, instead, a colema, which is a cross between a colonic and an enema. It is something you can perform yourself using some equipment and herbs which his book describes for you. He will tell you how and where to order them and how to use them. Dr. Jenson describes compacted, stringy, rubberized matter thirty inches long coming from the intestines after several colon cleanses. Proper eating, nutrition, and exercise can keep this build-up from occurring. However, most of us have abused our bodies for so many years, they need some special assistance to get back into normal operating condition.

If you don't want to use any special equipment but simply prefer utilizing some herbs and liquid clay to loosen compacted matter from the walls of your intestines, we will describe a fourteen-day program which does so in the chapter on fasting. **This will probably be the best place for a person to start.** People who start with this fourteen-day colon cleanse find that it is very seldom necessary to go beyond it to more advanced techniques. The developer of this fourteen-day herbal and clay cleanse is Dr. Albert Zehr, who was himself trained by Bernard Jenson. I talked to Dr. Zehr over the phone and asked him to compare the two approaches. He told me that he felt that 95 percent of the people would have their health needs met with the fourteen-day cleanse. However, they could then go on to the colema, if they feel a need. We have seen some dramatic results with the fourteen-day program.

One national beauty queen took enemas each morning in order to help keep her skin sparkling and energy high. Kind of amazing, isn't it?

We cannot have a healthy body without clean blood, and we cannot have clean blood unless we have a clean bowel with good tone to move wastes along promptly. A toxic bowel is the source of many health problems.

For Further Reading

Tissue Cleansing Through Bowel Management by Bernard Jenson D.C., Nutritionist.

Healthy Steps by Dr. Albert Zehr – Discusses fourteen-day colon cleanse using herbs, and a four-day fast in the middle of it. Also discusses many other interesting health approaches.

References

[1] Jensen, Bernard, *Tissue Cleansing Through Bowel Management* (Escondido, CA: Bernard Jensen Enterprises, 1981), p. A-5.

[2] Jensen, p. A-5.

[3] (clipping taken from the Daily News Service, 1981).

[4] Jensen, *Tissue Cleansing Through Bowel Management* p. 28.

[5] Jenson, p. 31.

[6] Jenson, p. 91.

Chapter 8

The Healing Value of Vitamins, Enzymes, Antioxidants and Herbs

"I will give no deadly drugs to anyone." Hippocrates

I don't know about you, but the statistics of the last several chapters make me think that everyone in the civilized world is bound to die through the continuous poisoning of the cells of their bodies. I really have had enough negative statistics to last me a lifetime. I could use some hope! Well, the great thing about the rest of this book is that it is filled with hope. It will show you many more things you can do to help your immune system stay strong, and make up for what is lacking in the impure land, impure food, and impure air.

Vitamins and the RDA

What fun we will have sorting out this sticky issue! Some claim that if you eat right, you don't need any vitamins. Others swear by them. Some say the RDA (Recommended Daily Allowance) is plenty. Others say it doesn't begin to meet our daily requirements for optimal health. Dr. McDougall's books, which we recommended in earlier chapters, suggest very strongly that you don't need supplements. Let's see what we can find out.

In California, it is against the law for a medical doctor to prescribe vitamins, and some medical doctors in California have been thrown in jail for doing so. That is quite an intense stand against vitamins.

I personally believe that because the land is so devitalized, the crops so covered with pesticides, and the air so filled with smog, it makes sense to supplement even a good diet with a few extra vitamins. Since we know that the cure comes from within, from our own immune system, we should be sure to give it all the supplies it needs to wage an aggressive, ongoing war. Vitamins, minerals, enzymes, amino acids, and other natural disciplines like fasting, exercise, rest and a positive mental attitude are the tools that our immune system needs for efficient operation.

Think of your body as approximately 70 trillion tiny little engines, which all work in harmony one with another. It is essential these engines have the right fuel so they can carry out their tasks. Vitamins work together with enzymes, as coenzymes, thereby allowing all the activities that occur within the body to happen quickly and accurately. Water-soluble vitamins (C and B complex) must be taken into the body daily, as they cannot be stored and are excreted within one to four days. Oil soluble vitamins (A,D,E,K) can be stored for longer periods of time.

The Recommended Daily Allowance (RDA) was instituted about forty years ago by the U.S. Food and Nutrition Board as a guide for preventing such diseases as scurvy, rickets, and night blindness. However, my goal in life is not to prevent scurvy in my body. My goal is to have **optimum** health and vitality. So I will look instead at another table which has been constructed, the **Optimum Daily Allowance (ODA).** A chart of the ODA can be found on page 11 of *Prescription for Nutritional Healing*, a comprehensive and up-to-date, self-help guide by James F. Balch, M.D. and Phyllis A. Balch, C.N.C. It is a practical A-to-Z reference to drug-free remedies using vitamins, minerals, herbs, amino acids, antioxidants, and natural food supplements, with 360 pages of health information that simply must be a part of your home health library.

For instance, I have heard for years that in order to fully absorb certain vitamins, I needed to take them in conjunction with other vitamins. I could never keep straight which ones went with which ones, or for that matter, which vitamin to take for certain ailments. On page 12 of the Balches' book, they provide a complete list of what vitamins to take in conjunction with others in order to achieve maximum benefits. And over 200 pages list various common disorders people have, and what vitamins, herbs, minerals and enzymes to take (in their proper order of importance) to give your immune system the tools it needs to effectively fight back and win. Wow! Not bad! It has become my nutritional bible. They even tell what the toxic limits are to each vitamin, as well as any other warnings which may apply.

Vitamins work best when taken with meals, because the nutrients in the meal make up anything that is needed for complete assimilation of the vitamin.

You should always take natural vitamins, not synthetic or chemical vitamins. Synthetic vitamins are produced in a laboratory from isolated chemicals that mirror their counterparts found in nature. They may have in them coal tars, artificial coloring, preservatives, sugars, starch, and other additives. Their value is only a fraction of that of a similar natural vitamin, and they can be dangerous.

Even though the RDA is not designed to give you maximum health, but only keep you from scurvy and the like, surveys reveal that **less than half** of the population take in even the RDA. That is scary. That means one-half of us are not even getting enough vitamins to keep us from scurvy! According to U.S. Senate Document No. 264, 99 percent of Americans are deficient in minerals. The World Health Organization ranks the top 42 nations of the world for their nutritional diets. America ranks as the 38th best fed country in the world (OUT OF 42!!!). How is this possible? Of the approximately 12,000 food items in a well-stocked grocery store, 80 percent have been processed (i.e. tampered with by man).

A poll of 37,000 people, conducted by Food Technology (1981), indicated that half of the population was deficient in vitamin B6, 42 percent did not consume sufficient amounts of calcium, 39 percent had an insufficient iron intake, and 25 to 39 percent did not obtain the needed amounts of vitamin C. And the RDA amount of vitamin C is only 60 mg, whereas hundreds of studies have shown that the optimum amount of Vitamin C is in the range of 5000 mg to 12,000 mg per day.

The American Dietetic Association, which is the professional organization of registered dietitians, will tell you that you can get everything you need from the food you eat, and you do not need to supplement your diet. On the other hand, sixty percent of its members take food supplements. **That is more than twice the percentage of average Americans who take food supplements!** So the organization's party line is, "You don't need them", but sixty percent of its members take them. Do you suppose they know something they are not telling us? Of course the Bible says that one way to discover what a person really believes is to examine the fruit in his life — what he actually does, not what he says he believes.

Because I don't (and sometimes can't) eat properly all the time, I decided to regularly take a good, natural vitamin, mineral and calcium supplement. I found one which is bonded to fructose (a natural sugar which your cells love) and thus is **completely** assimilated by your body. Do not go to the pharmacy and buy synthetic vitamins. Their value is limited. According to law, if the vitamin is made of 10 to 15 percent natural ingredients, it can claim to be natural. Buy vitamins which are listed as **completely** natural, not just natural, for optimum benefit.

One study by Dr. Henry Ogle of Crest Hill, Illinois compared the amount of vitamin E found in the blood one hour after taking vitamin E supplements. A synthetic brand released .75 percent. The average health food store brand released 3.5 percent, while the best health store brand released 15 percent. However, an all-natural direct mail order brand released 90 percent. All vitamins are not created equal.

To help answer the question as to how much better natural vitamins might be to synthetic vitamins, Dr. Graham Burton, a Canadian researcher of the National Research Council of Canada, gave equal doses of both natural and synthetic vitamin E to experimental animals, and then measured the proportion of both types of vitamin E in various organs, tissues, and fluids of his subjects. In the brains of mice, for example, Burton found 5.3 times more natural vitamin E than the synthetic variety. Burton therefore concluded that the body prefers natural vitamin E to synthetic vitamin E.

Why is it so important that the ingredient begins showing up in the blood within one hour? According to testing standards set by Howard University's School of Pharmacy, based on governmentally mandated tests used for pharmaceuticals, uncoated tablets must disintegrate within thirty minutes and coated tablets in one hour in order for nutrients to be absorbed into the system. I did an experiment with the natural multi-vitamin and calcium supplements I take. I put them in a glass of water and within thirty minutes they had dissolved. Great! In addition, the brand I take bonds the vitamins to fructose on the molecular level, so they are completely assimilated by my cells. Make sure that what you are taking does dissolve and does get assimilated. Do some testing. Know for sure. Don't just hope. Make sure your efforts toward health are not being wasted. Some vitamins take four hours to dissolve. Some never do.

If you are going to be completely vegetarian (which I am not personally doing), you need to supplement your diet with B_{12} as this vitamin is essential in keeping one from becoming anemic. It is normally found in such foods as cheese, clams, eggs, liver, mackerel, mild seafood and Tofu, but is not found in vegetables. It is available only from animal sources. One lady friend of ours went strictly vegetarian for a year with no meats and no dairy product and ended up extremely anemic, with very low hemoglobin numbers, and immediately consumed large doses of B_{12} to get back into balance. Dr. James Balch, M.D. recommends 300mcg of B_{12} per day to maintain excellent health.

Enzymes

It has often been said that you are not what you eat, but rather what you absorb of your diet. Enzymes are what allow your body to absorb the food you take in. Enzymes are found in all living plant and animal matter and are essential for maintaining proper functioning of the body, digesting food, and aiding in the repair of tissue. The body cannot be sustained without enzymes. The body creates its own enzymes, as well as receiving enzymes from the food we eat. However, enzymes are extremely sensitive to heat and begin to die at 107 degrees. They are totally dead at 120 degrees. All heated and processed food, as well as all cooked food, has been depleted of all enzymes. If you are not taking in a fair amount of raw food, you are putting an extra strain on your body. This overuse can impair the functioning capacity of the body, making it susceptible to cancer, obesity, cardiovascular disease, and a host of other illnesses.

Fortunately, enzymes can be purchased in capsule form and taken as a supplement along with your meal. This can help make up what is lacking in one's diet. I have found it very easy to simply add an enzyme capsule to my daily diet.

Herbs

My introduction to herbs is actually quite an interesting story. It began with a phone call to Lance, a pastor and friend of mine from Rhode Island. As we chatted, he spoke of a natural food supplement, in capsule form, which he and his wife had begun taking three months earlier. It had increased their metabolic rate, causing each of them to lose fifteen pounds, while at the same time increasing their energy. Many people in their church had seen the difference in their lives and were beating a track to their door, wanting to purchase whatever it was they were taking.

Piqued Interest

Well, I was intrigued enough to say, "Send me a sample and I will see if it works for me." As you may know, I could never be classified as skinny. I didn't really think much would happen because I have tried many things like this, and they have never worked, but since "hope never fails," I will try anything anyone wants to send me. If it doesn't work, I haven't lost anything. If it does work, I could actually end up thinner and with more energy.

Startling Results

Well, it worked! Unbelievable! This product actually did what it was advertised to do. I lost four inches around my waist in the first five weeks. I have never in my life lost so much, and I was not even dieting. I was just taking two capsules of this product each day. The other wonderful thing was that it restored my energy level to that of twenty years ago, when I was only twenty years of age! Talk about ecstatic! Within two months, I had lost six inches from my waist plus inches around my neck, hips, and thighs. My eating habits were altered some- what because I no longer craved sweets and junk food. From October 14, 1993 to January 17, 1994, the records in my doctor's office show that my cholesterol dropped from 272 to 209, a 63-point drop in three months. That constitutes a 500 percent lower chance of coronary problems! Wow!

Background

Before I began taking this product, I would eat a meal and feel stuffed, yet still have low energy. I would have a craving to eat more to try to get my energy up. I knew my body was not working right, but I had no idea how to fix it, or what was wrong. Now that I am taking these herbs, I find that at the close of a meal I have not eaten as much because my appetite has been curbed; plus, I feel energy and no desire to continue eating. Something had adjusted me internally. What was it?

Eleven Healing Herbs

Of course, I had begun to study the eleven herbs and chromium picolinate which are in the capsule. I began my investigation by showing a list of the herbs to my naturopath, Dr. Michael A. Prytula, MD (who specializes in herbs), to make sure they were not dangerous and would do as advertised.

Dr. Prytula assured me that the herbs were not dangerous, and that they would indeed do exactly what the company brochures claimed they would do. He suggested taking them for two months, then giving my body a rest by not taking them for one month. These herbs were a great way to **kick start** my body into energy and life again. I used the energy and life which I received to study and personally apply the good principles of diet and health care which are recorded in this book. May I suggest that this approach could be helpful to others also.

Even the Bible says:

"He causeth the grass to grow for the cattle and **herbs** for the service of humanity" (Psalms 104:14 KJV).

I must have missed this verse in my earlier Biblical studies. It is amazing how much of the Bible I don't see until I first experience the truth myself. Then, when I go back and read it again, I see the truth was there all the time. And to think that I have tended to relegate God's wonderful gift of healing herbs to either the New Age movement or earlier, less sophisticated, times. Just because I am not living a particular verse, why must I consign it to either the evil or the uninformed? Perhaps I have a problem that needs to be taken to the cross. Maybe that is why I should walk in meekness rather than thinking I know so much. Maybe I remain mostly blind until life's experiences and God's revelation and God's Word converge upon me. Only then do I "see".

This was my first introduction to a study of herbs. I have since purchased a book entitled The Healing Herbs, and found that these herbs have been used and listed in herb dictionaries for thousands of years. As a matter of fact, they will do far more than the one line descriptions given above, and they are much more widely used in Europe by the medical practice than in America. (Europe allows a much wider range of medicines to be practiced than does America. The American Medical Regulatory Agencies are, at this point in American history, quite narrow in focus, and dictatorial in approach. It is time for some servants to take positions of leadership and guide our nation and medical profession into the truth of God's words and ways. I wonder if we, you and I, should be these new leaders. I suspect so. I promise I will strive with you to become a servant leader in as many areas as God allows me to stretch and grow.)

Scientific studies showing the benefits of some of these herbs have appeared in the British Medical Journal Lancet and the New England Journal of Medicine. Products made from ginko are among Europe's most widely prescribed medications, with sales of $500 million a year.[1] I recommend that those wanting a more detailed description of the research done on the healing properties of these herbs purchase the book *The Healing Herbs* by Michael Castleman.

Chromium Picolinate

The other ingredient in the product I tried is chromium picolinate, so my next area of research was to study about that (U.S. patent # 4,315,927).

The information below is drawn and condensed from a fascinating booklet entitled *Chromium Picolinate* (a part of the *Good Health Guide Series*) written by Richard A. Passwater, Ph.D. I highly recommend that you purchase and study a copy of the booklet. It contains forty-eight pages of scientific research backing up the following claims about chromium picolinate. I am excerpting just a few of these studies for your consideration. (Picolinate may be pronounced either "pick-o-LIN-ate" or "pie-COL-lin-ate.")

An insulin co-factor

Chromium picolinate is an essential insulin co-factor. The hormone insulin helps control hunger and regulates energy production, fat burning, muscle building, and cholesterol utilization. Insulin is like a doorkeeper that controls the passage of nutrients and other important compounds through the walls of your 70 trillion body cells.

Americans have inadequate amounts of chromium

Ninety percent of U.S. diets are below the lowest level of the recommended daily chromium intake. Food processing removes up to 80 percent of the chromium of many whole foods. Consumption of high-sugar diets increases chromium excretion by 10 to 300 percent. Asians have four to five times more chromium in their bodies than Americans.

Losing excess body fat while gaining muscle

Chromium picolinate promotes permanent fat loss because it normalizes metabolism. It will produce a gradual but steady and persistent loss of body fat. When chromium is complimented as it should be with a reduction in dietary fat and an increase in exercise, the fat loss is proportionally accelerated. (Note: One person I introduced to this product also cut fat from his diet and lost thirty pounds in one month).

One study was done at a prominent weight-loss clinic in San Antonio, Texas under the direction of Dr. Gilbert Kaats. Volunteers consumed two nutritional drinks each day and were asked not to change their food intake or exercise activity. Some of the drinks contained no chromium picolinate, some 200 micrograms of chromium picolinate and others 400 micrograms. Neither the doctors nor the volunteers knew how much chromium picolinate was in the drinks until after the study. Others had prepared the drinks, coded them, and kept the codes secret until after the study. Then the code was released and the results compiled.

After seventy-two days, the group receiving no chromium picolinate had essentially no fat loss or muscle gain. However, the groups receiving chromium picolinate lost an average of 4.2 pounds of fat, and gained an average of 1.4 pounds of muscle. That is a net improvement of 5.6 pounds, for a net enhancement of the physique.

Results were best in the older volunteers, which is not surprising as chromium deficiency increases with age. Those taking 400 micrograms of chromium picolinate daily averaged a 27 percent better response than those taking 200 micrograms.

Scientists at Louisiana State University, searching for a way to grow lean pork naturally, tested chromium picolinate on pigs. They found that chromium picolinate reduced fat measured at the tenth rib by 21 percent and increased muscle 7 percent.

Chromium picolinate appears to stoke up the metabolic rate

In typical dieting, both fat and lean muscle are lost. Then, when weight is put back on, a greater proportion tends to be fat and a lesser proportion, muscle, leaving the person "fatter" than ever. However, when losing weight with chromium picolinate, fat is lost while muscle is being gained. Therefore one's "shape" is being restored. Even though this will take place without exercising, it takes place even more readily if exercise and chromium are coupled together. I think this was my experience because my scales showed that I had only lost three pounds, even though my waist had decreased by four inches. I suspect I had lost fat and gained muscle weight, which is fine with me. I had been exercising for twenty minutes a day for six months before I began taking these herbs and chromium. However, I was not seeing the change in shape or increase in energy I normally had achieved in my younger years as a result of exercise. I suspect this was because, now that I am older, the chromium was more depleted in my body.

Good news — dieting is dead!

In October 1993, Prevention magazine ran an article entitled "Good News: Dieting is Dead" (p. 39ff). Tufts University in Boston took a group of men and woman in their 60's and divided them into an exercise group and a diet group. The exercise group worked out twice a day on a stationary bike, burning 360 calories but eating exactly the same number of calories as they were eating before the 12-week program began. The diet group ate exactly 360 calories a day less than they had been eating before. The diet group lost eleven pounds and the exercise group, sixteen pounds. However, six pounds lost by the diet group was muscle and only five pounds was fat. The exercise group actually gained three pounds of pure muscle; so, in reality, they lost nineteen pounds of fat, or four times more fat than the dieters.

Lowering Cholesterol

Studies show that if blood levels of chromium reach optimal levels, heart disease is extremely unlikely. In addition, chromium can eradicate existing cholesterol deposits in the arteries. Chromium increases HDL production, according to one study, by 17 to 23 percent and reduces total cholesterol by 10 to 36 percent. HDL are the scavengers which take excess cholesterol out of one's system and dump it in the liver. Once this increased number of HDL scavengers removes excess cholesterol from the bloodstream, they begin cleaning and stripping some of the cholesterol from deposits in the arteries.

In one study, patients proven to have coronary blockage had an average plasma-chromium level of 1.05 mcg/liter; in those without coronary blockage, it was 8.51 mcg/liter.

Preventing and controlling diabetes and hypoglycemia

Diabetes is a condition in which there is an insulin problem. In the 1950's, when healthy laboratory rats were fed a chromium-deficient diet, they developed the symptoms of diabetes. When they were properly nourished with chromium, these symptoms quickly disappeared.

Chromium picolinate reduces high blood sugar

One group of researchers at the Mercy Hospital and Medical Center of San Diego found that 200 micrograms of chromium picolinate reduced fasting blood sugar levels by 18 percent and glycosylated hemoglobin levels by 10 percent in just six weeks.

Strengthening the immune system and increasing lifespan

In one study, which was looking for signs of chromium toxicity, the researchers discovered that the more chromium they fed the laboratory animals, the longer they seemed to live. After thirty months, almost half of the laboratory rats (nine of twenty) in the groups fed 0-2.08 micrograms of chromium picolinate per gram of diet had died, while only one rat (of thirty) had died in the groups given 4.2-42 micrograms of chromium picolinate per gram of diet.

Researchers have been not able to get enough chromium picolinate into laboratory animals to produce any adverse effects. Their estimation of the toxic level is in excess of 2.2 grams per kilogram of body weight, which is equivalent to 156,000 milligrams for a 154 pound person.

For further study

The above is only bits and pieces of a few of many studies cited in the booklet *Chromium Picolinate* by Richard A. Passwater, Ph.D. I highly recommend you purchase and study his entire booklet.

I have decided to take these herbs and chromium as a regular part of my diet, and I highly recommend it as an all-natural nutritional supplement that will make one look better, feel better, and have more energy. I do encourage you to follow my naturopath's recommendation of two months on, one month off.

Antioxidants

An antioxidant helps destroy free radicals in one's body. Free radicals have been shown to be major contributors to more than sixty of our major diseases. The "Mayo Clinic Health Letter" (August 1993) had the following diagram and quote on its front page:

The following brief overview is taken from the booklet *The Antioxidants* by Richard A. Passwater, Ph.D. I highly recommend you purchase this booklet. It is part of *The Good Health Guide Series*.

Antioxidants are nutrients that guard your body against cancer, heart disease, arthritis, allergies, cataracts, and even slow the aging process. The antioxidants we will study are vitamin A (beta carotene), selenium, vitamin E, vitamin C.

A free radical is highly reactive because its electron arrangement is out of "spin" balance. Each free radical is capable of destroying an enzyme or protein molecule or even an entire cell. Each free radical

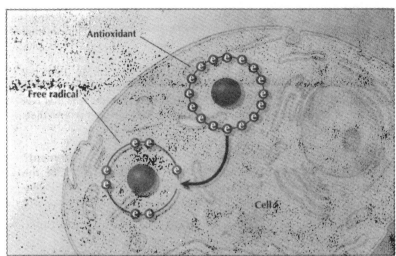

Artwork courtesy of *Mayo Clinic Health Letter* with permission of Mayo Foundation for Medical Education and Research, Rochester, Minnesota 55905.

"A free radical is a damaged molecule with a missing electron. An antioxidant, such as vitamin C, vitamin E, or beta carotene, may donate one of its electrons to the free radical. If an antioxidant doesn't 'help', a free radical takes an electron from vital cell structures, damaging the cell and eventually leading to disease."

usually generates a chain of free-radical reactions, resulting in thousands of free radicals being released to destroy body components.

Cancer and Vitamin A

A healthy body can overcome cancer, just as it can ward off cancer. In one of Dr. Umberto Saffioti's experiments when he was at the Chicago Medical School, 113 hamsters were dosed with the cigarette smoke carcinogen benzopyrene. Of the 53 control animals not given extra vitamin A protection, 16 developed lung cancer. However, of the 60 vitamin A-treated animals, only one developed lung cancer and four developed benign tumors. Dr. E. Bjelke of the Cancer Registry of Norway found that 74 percent of the men with lung cancer were in the lowest third of the population, ranked by vitamin A intake. Vitamin A-deficient city dwellers have three times the lung cancer rate of better-nourished city dwellers. Similarly, Dr. Richard Doll, president of the British Association for Cancer Research, found that beta carotene reduced cancer incidence in laboratory animals by 40 percent.

Selenium

Dr. Gerhard Schrauzer, of the University of California at San Diego, found that dietary selenium reduced the incidence of cancer in a strain of mice to only 10 percent. They normally have an 80 to 85 percent incidence of breast cancer due to a virus they ingest with their mother's milk. In addition, among those that did develop cancer, the disease did not appear until 50 percent later than among the control animals, and the tumors were less malignant. Rapid City, South Dakota has the lowest cancer rate of any city in the United States, and the citizens of Rapid City also have the highest measured blood selenium levels in the nation. But in Lima, Ohio, which has twice the cancer rate of Rapid City, the citizens have only 60 percent of the blood selenium levels of those in Rapid City.

Vitamin E

Vitamin E has been shown to help prevent cancers caused by many chemicals in our environment. This is important because scientists estimate that 80 to 95 percent of human cancers are caused by environmental carcinogens.

Vitamin C

A Cameron-Pauling study compared one hundred terminally ill patients given 10,000 milligrams of vitamin C per day to 1000 other such patients. Both groups were treated identically in all ways — by the same physicians in the same hospital — except one was not given the vitamin C. At the time the study report was prepared, those patients given vitamin C had lived more than four times longer than the matched "control" patients. The patient survival rate continued to improve long after the report was published.

Dr. Pauling, from the Mayo Clinic, estimates "that with proper use of vitamin C for cancer, we could cut the death rate by 75% of the 360,000 people who die every year of cancer." Vitamin C also reduces the patients' pain and improves their sense of well-being, appetite, and mental alertness.

(Note: The Mayo Clinic (Creagan 1979) found only a small protective effect of vitamin C. Dr. Ewan Cameron criticized this study as being so flawed that the conclusion cannot be accepted. Highlights of his criticism are found on page xx of Cancer and Vitamin C.

A second flawed study appeared in the New England Journal, April 14, 1994 and received widespread media coverage. This study concluded that vitamin E and beta carotene were not helpful in preventing cancer in long-term smokers, and in fact, apparently caused cancer, since a slight increase in cancer was observed. Problems with this study include the following: 1) It was carried out only on long-term smokers (average thirty-six years of smoking), who did not stop smoking but averaged twenty cigarettes per day; 2) The more potent antioxidant, vitamin C, was curiously absent from the study. Numerous studies have shown that the interaction of all the known antioxidants confer benefit; 3) Participants were given either beta carotene OR vitamin E, not both. The amount of beta carotene was pitifully inadequate — 20 milligrams per day. 4) Also, both smoking and drinking reduce the blood levels of beta carotene by 20 percent. This group not only smoked an average of twenty cigarettes per day, they also drank an average of 10.9 grams of alcohol a day. Wouldn't it have been nice if the newspapers had told the public "the rest of the story"? I wonder why they didn't.

(It takes real sensitivity and discernment to discover truth. I guess we just need to walk humbly and say, "This is as much of the truth as I can discern at this point in my life.")

In 1973, the Norwegian Cancer Registry's researcher, Dr. Bjelke, surveyed 30,000 people and found that the greater the intake of vitamin C, the smaller the incidence of cancer.

Synergy

Combinations of antioxidants provide better protection than might be expected when considering each antioxidant individually; the effect is synergistic, an example of the whole being greater than the sum of its parts. So taking combinations of vitamins A, C, and E, plus the trace mineral selenium, is more effective than larger amounts of the individual antioxidant nutrients.

Aging

Aging is the process that reduces the number of healthy cells in the body. Antioxidants slow the aging process. Dr. Passwater found in his experiments with laboratory animals that their lifespans were increased by 175 percent by consuming antioxidants.

Heart Disease and Vitamin E

Antioxidant nutrients help prevent heart disease by protecting the arteries against the damage that leads to the cholesterol deposits called plaque, but the risk of heart attacks is more significantly decreased by

the nutrients' ability to keep fatal blood clots from form
coronary arteries.

In one study of 17,894 people, the amount of heart disease in any
age group decreased proportionately with the length of time the participants took vitamin E. One group consisted of those who had taken
400 IU or more of vitamin E daily for at least ten years. The study
included 2,508 such people between the ages of 50 and 98. Based on
Department of Health, Education and Welfare figures (HRS 74-
1222,1976), normally 836 of the 2,508 would be expected to have heart
disease. Instead, there were only four. This is less than one percent of
the expected number.

Arthritis

The pain, swelling, and inflammation of arthritis are also caused by
free radicals. Human studies in Great Britain have found that approximately 80 percent of arthritis sufferers found significant relief from
pain, and reduced swelling and inflammation, by taking the combination of antioxidant nutrients, vitamins A, C, and E, plus the trace
mineral selenium. Researchers have found that rheumatoid arthritis
patients have lower than normal levels of selenium in their blood.

Cataracts

Antioxidant levels in a cataracted lens are a fraction of those in a
healthy lens. Several researchers have found that they can slow or halt
the growth of cataracts by having their patients take supplements of
the antioxidant nutrients, thus normalizing the antioxidant levels of
the lens.

Allergies

Chemical hypersensitivities are often caused by free-radical reactions. Many people who are allergic (sensitive) to various chemicals
have found that their allergies disappeared soon after taking antioxidant nutrients.

In Summary

The above is only a brief summary of a few studies which are
reviewed in *The Antioxidants* by Richard A. Passwater, Ph.D. I recommend you purchase this booklet.

I have decided that antioxidants represent the best preventive medicine I have discovered, to date, to keep me from many of life's threatening diseases. Unfortunately, modern medicine has focused on cures for sicknesses rather than ways of preventing them. Personally, I would rather prevent them. Antioxidants are one of the means I can use to do so.

Unfortunately, of the $900 billion spent annually in the area of medicine, almost all is spent on attempts to cure disease rather than prevention, and half is spent in the last three months before death!

It has amazed me that modern Western medicine has done so poorly in finding solutions for cancer, heart disease, and other degenerative diseases. Their solution has been to cut us open and take out the parts that are diseased, and then radiate what is left, killing off even more of us. And this is after they have spent billions of dollars in research over a fifty-year period. Their best estimates now are that by the year 2000, 41 percent of Americans will contract cancer in their lifetimes, and be cut and radiated in a painful and costly attempt to add a few meager years to one's life. Isn't that a refreshing statistic? The solutions I have found in my research and offered in this book may seem radical and costly at first. But when compared to the alternatives, they don't really seem so bad after all, do they?

What about the safety of vitamins and herbs?

According to the "Townsend Letter for Doctors", the number of deaths reported to the Poison Control Center in 1991 related to pharmaceuticals was 9,805. The number of deaths caused by vitamins, herbs, minerals, and amino acids was "0". That should really tell us a lot! As a matter of fact, Dr. Julian Whitaker stated that there have been no reported deaths due to vitamins or minerals in the last ten years. Apparently, there is a much smaller likelihood of hurting yourself with these than with pharmaceutical medicines.

According to the National Center for Health Statistics, in the Mortality Report of the U.S. 1989, 180 people per 100,000 die from medicaments every year. Based on 250 million people in this country, that means that modern medicine, specifically pharmaceutical drugs, kills 450,000 Americans every year. In addition, according to the General Accounting Office, as of the early 1970's, there were over six million adverse reactions to prescription drugs annually. If a natural medicine, which was unable to be patented and thus merchandised, killed even twenty- five people, it would be banned from sale by the FDA. Why does the FDA allow 450,000 deaths per year from patentable, merchandisable, synthetic, pharmaceutical products without requiring that they be taken off the market? Could this be a double standard?

God's covenant of health through herbs

"And he cried unto the LORD; and the LORD showed him a tree, which when he had cast into the waters, the waters were made sweet: there He made for them a statute and an ordinance, and there He proved them, And said, If thou wilt diligently hearken to the voice of the LORD thy God, and wilt do that which is right in His sight, and wilt give ear to His commandments, and keep all His statutes, I will put none of these diseases upon thee, which I have brought upon the Egyptians: for I am the LORD that healeth thee (literally 'is your health')" (Exodus 15:25,26).

It is interesting that when God gave Israel the Covenant of Health, **it was not actually connected with a power miracle. It was connected with a miracle of knowledge** (word of knowledge), as God showed Moses a tree which he could put into the bitter water to make it sweet. Is God saying that if we will let Him give us wisdom concerning which herbs to use, He will show us a way of living in health? It appears so to me.

Why do herbs heal?

So what is so great about the bark and roots of trees that they (herbs) heal us? The answer is in the fact that bark and roots are anti-fungal and anti-bacterial because they were designed to ward off insects. As a result, they have healing capabilities in our bodies.

Pycnogenol — the super antioxidant from the bark of the French Maritime Pine

Pycnogenol has been shown in clinical studies to be twenty times more effective than vitamin C and fifty times more effective than vitamin E as an antioxidant. In fact, pycnogenol appears to be the most powerful antioxidant ever discovered. It is anti-inflammatory, antihistamine, strengthens blood vessels, acts against gum bleeding, and much more. The stories told by one doctor of its healing power make me picture pycnogenol as a "super-smart missile" which, when consumed in capsule form, goes into your body and targets any damaged cells, restoring them. He even told of it dissolving inoperable, cancerous tumors. If I were struggling with cancer, I would certainly be trying it. As a matter of fact, I am taking pycnogenol simply as a preventive measure. An ounce of prevention....

My secretary had torn her knee internally in a skiing accident, and it had left her with ongoing pain whenever she tried to exercise. After taking a saturation dosage of pycnogenol, she was out and running three miles a day with no pain. If you have any cellular damage in your body, you can't lose anything by giving pycnogenol a try for three weeks. If it is going to work, you will know by then and, if not, you can discontinue its use. As a matter of fact, I think anything that is going to work ought to do so within three weeks to three months. If I have not experienced anything by that time, I discontinue its use. Listen to your body.

On the other hand, some things are taken not to heal a problem but to **prevent** a problem from occurring, such as antioxidants. In such situations I may not **feel** any better, since I wasn't sick in the first place. I take them in faith believing they are doing their preventive work.

Aloe Vera — Miracle Healing Plant

You may know of aloe as an external lotion with an amazing capacity to heal burns and cuts. However, did you know aloe can be taken internally also, for internal healing purposes? I have a video with H. Reginald McDaniel, M.D. and several AIDS patients who were healed while under his care. One patient shown on the video was Michael Arrington, who had been given four to twenty days to live, and had seventeen malignant tumors in his liver, one the size of a baseball. His X-rays clearly showed the tumors on the video. Six months after starting on aloe vera, the tumors were completely gone, and he was not on any other medicines. His doctor, H. Reginald McDaniel, showed X-rays after the healing. All tumors were gone. He also showed X-rays of a lady with breast cancer whose cancer disappeared after drinking aloe vera. Dr. McDaniel's conclusion is, "The use of aloe vera will be the most important single step forward in the treatment of diseases in the history of mankind."

Essentially, aloe **builds the immune system,** so it helps you ward off all disease, including cancer and AIDS.

However, do beware, because many aloe drinks have been tested and found to be incredibly weak, and some border on absolute fraud. The healing agent in aloe is mucopolysaccharides (MEOH). For a fee of about $75, North Texas Research Laboratory in Grand Prairie,

Texas (214-263-1059) will test a sample of aloe for you to see how much MEOH it actually contains. In the appendix of *Aloe Vera: A Mission Discovered*, Lee Ritter lists the test results of many aloe products he has tested. (See appendix of this book for a reprint of these test results.)

We sent some aloe to North Texas Research Laboratory for testing and received some interesting results. I am involved with two companies which make aloe available for internal use, one as a liquid, one in capsule form. In testing these two, we discovered that one bottle of **90 capsules** of aloe was equivalent, in MEOH concentration, to **64 liters** of aloe liquid by the other company. So don't just buy any aloe. Know what you are getting.

Only a Sampling

The list above of God's amazing miracle cures is only a sampling of many, many cures you will want to search out over the years. These are simply some of the ones I have found that have proven effective, and so I pass them on to you. May I suggest that you enjoy a number of years of personal exploration and discovery and share the wonder of the world in which God has placed us.

Books for Further Study

Prescription for Nutritional Healing by James F. Balch, M.D. and Phyllis A. Balch, C.N.C.

Digestive Enzymes by Jeffrey Bland, Ph.D.

The Antioxidants by Dr. Richard Passwater.

Chromium Picolinate by Dr. Richard Passwater.

The New Superantioxidant-Plus (Pycnogenol) by Dr. Richard Passwater.

Free Radicals and Disease Prevention by David J. Lin – an illustrated, easy to read introduction to free radicals and disease prevention. Filled with statistics. Down-to-earth. Very good.

The Healing Herbs by Michael Castleman – contains remedies for over 200 conditions and diseases.

Aloe Vera: A Mission Discovered by Lee Ritter – 176 pages of information about aloe vera.

Healthy Steps by Albert Zehr, Ph.D. – 154 pages on the use of combinations of herbs, vitamins, and antioxidants to heal various common problems. He also works in conjunction with a company that markets these combinations. For those interested, the herb combinations which they sell are as follows.

Product Combinations:
1 — Gastro-Intestinal Problems
2 — Internal Cleansing - Detoxification Formula
3 — Respiratory Ailments
4 — Female Complaints and Female Irregularities
5 — Nervous Conditions and Relaxation
6 — Kidney Ailments
7 — Eliminate Parasites or Worms
8 — Blood Sugar Levels
9 — Reduce Fever
10 — Flu symptom
11 — Male Irregularities
12 — Depress the Appetite

If I had any of the above problems, I would rather go to herbs which would build my immune system and cure me naturally than to synthetic medicines which tend to poison my body and damage it, leaving it with many harmful side effects. If you are not aware of the harmful side effects of a drug which your doctor is prescribing, ask to look at his copy of *The Physician's Desk Reference*. Let him show you the pages which deal with that particular drug. You might even want to photocopy the pages for further study. It may convince you to try something natural first. These combinations have been carefully researched and on the market doing their healing work for years. They are not going to hurt you. Trying them for a few weeks may give you a pleasant surprise. If not, nothing will have been lost in your experiment. My belief is that the herbs which God has given for the healing of mankind (Ps. 104:14) will work better than man's synthetic approach.

References

[1] Castleman, Michael, *The Healing Herbs* (Emmaus, PA: Rodale Press, 1991), p. 190.

Chapter 9

The Healing Value
of Exercise

Empowering For the Body

Even though health authorities have been telling us since the 1970's that we should exercise for our health, nearly four out of five adults get little or no exercise, according to the Centers for Disease Control. A friend of mine, Rev. Mike Bickle, has the perfect solution. He told me that since his wife exercises and the two of them are "one", she covers the exercise quota for him also. Cute!

I was one of those who fell in love with jogging 25 years ago (Shudder! It's hard to believe it could be that long!), and I have jogged about a mile and a half, three to five days a week, rather continuously for the last 25 years.

I do it because **I love it!** I love the feeling I get emotionally. Those endorphins (anti-depressants) are released and my body loves the feeling! I also love the mental clarity it gives me. I feel sharp all morning after I have exercised. And jogging has kept me from turning into a blob of fat, which is the definite tendency that my body moves toward.

However, I had made the wrong assumption that aerobic exercise was all I needed, and I have suffered a penalty for that. I did not realize that stretching exercises are also important or your muscles become tighter (especially as you get older — which I am **not** doing) and begin to pull your body out of joint. The consequence of this lack of knowl-edge in my life has been regular trips to the chiropractor, about every two to three months, to have my lower back put back in place. This, I have discovered, can be avoided (or at least greatly reduced) by regular stretching exercises.

So, let's talk for awhile about the healing value of exercise and the types of exercises we should all do. It does not take much exercise (twenty minutes, three to five days a week), and it does not need to be painful to give you tremendous value. And it doesn't need to be jogging. Many exercises increase your health and vitality, including walking, swimming, dancing and cycling, to name a few. The important thing is that out of the hundreds of exercises available, you choose one you like.

As a matter of fact, research has shown that just a very little exercise helps **a lot**. "For example, researchers from the Cooper Institute for Aerobics Research in Dallas gauged fitness in about 13,000 men and women by measuring how long the volunteers could exercise on a treadmill. Then, the researchers followed them for an average of more than eight years. As fitness increased, the death rate fell. But by far, the **biggest drop in mortality** — 60 percent for men, nearly 50 percent for the women — occurred between the most unfit volunteers and those who were just slightly more fit."[1]

Now isn't that refreshing to know? You don't have to do a lot of exercise, nor does it have to be strenuous exercise, in order to reap a tremendous health response. Essentially, it has been discovered that light exercise (two brisk 35-minute walks per week, for example) offers the greatest jump in improved health. Increasing to moderate exercise three to five days per week provides somewhat better health benefits, but very intense exercise can begin to produce some negative results. So, a little goes a long way, a moderate amount is best, and the most tiring is probably best avoided.

Exercise Stimulates Your Body's Healing Abilities!

Studies show that exercisers pay half as much in medical bills each year as do non-exercisers and have only one-third the number of sick days.[2]

Exercise burns away excess weight, lowers blood pressure, improves the cholesterol profile, improves blood sugar and insulin dynamics, helps prevent bone-thinning osteoporosis, helps alleviate chronic lower back pain, and improves immune function, mood and mental performance.

The Centers for Disease Control have performed two large studies which pinpoint exercise as the number one deficiency of Americans. If you do not get any exercise, your chances of having a heart attack are more than tripled, according to studies from the University of North Carolina at Chapel Hill. The Chapel Hill researchers stated that an inactive person's risk of heart disease is the same as that of someone **who smokes a pack of cigarettes a day** [emphasis mine].[3]

Physical Benefits of Exercise

1. Increases general bodily performance and agility

Some 4,500 people between ages 40 and 85 were studied at Brown University by Vincent Mor, PH.D. He concluded that people who remain physically active throughout their later years can gain as much as a 25 year advantage in performance over those who retire to their easy chairs. And moderate activity, such as walking, was all that was needed to keep these people agile.[4]

2. Lowers death rate from all diseases

16,936 Harvard alumni have been tracked for many years. It has been found that those men who burned 2,000 or more calories a week in exercise had a 28 percent lower death rate than men who exercised less or not at all. Ralph Paffenberger Jr., M.D., Ph.D., one of the authors of this study, stated, "...for every hour you walk, you can add an hour to your life."[5]

3. Reduces risk of cancer

In a study comprising 5000 female graduate students from 1925 to 1981, scientists at Harvard University found that less active women had a two-and-one-half times greater risk of developing cancer than did the former athletes among them. The sedentary group had twice the risk for breast cancer, as well as two to four times more cancer of the uterus, ovaries, cervix, and vagina.

4. Reduces risk of heart disease

A major study involving over 12,000 men who were at risk for developing heart disease was done at the University of Minnesota School of Public Health. The researchers spent seven years monitoring the men and found that the men who were least active had a 30 percent greater chance of death from heart attacks than moderately active men.

5. Lowers blood pressure

Dr. Martin put nineteen sedentary men with mild hypertension (high blood pressure) on a ten-week mild aerobic exercise program. The blood pressure in the group went from an average of 137/95 to 130/85.

6. Reduces back pain and back problems

Walking can be a wonderful preventive and curative of the most common kinds of muscular backache. "Even some cases of back pain where a disk problem has been identified will respond well to regular, rhythmic walking — three to six days a week, for 30 to 60 minutes per session."[6]

In an informal poll of 492 people with a variety of back problems, published in 1985, 98 percent of those who made walking a part of their regular routine found it helpful.[7]

Emotional benefits of exercise

1. It is an anti-depressant.

A doctoral thesis that reviewed seventy-seven studies concluded that depression exits the body along with sweat. "In fact," wrote Thomas Christian North, Ph.D., "exercise appears to be a better anti-depressant than psychological treatment."[8]

Another analysis of 81 different studies found that in 70 percent of the studies, significant improvement in mental state was associated with fitness.[8]

When you exercise, endorphins (anti-depressants) are released into your body and you experience a sense of well-being. It has been called the "runners high", but all aerobic exercise causes this wonderful sensation. It will last for several hours.

2. It allows you to handle stress more effectively.

"Both fit and unfit people were subjected to the mental stress of an arithmetic test. Meanwhile, researchers at the University of Toronto monitored both the rate and the electrical activity of their hearts.

"'Even with this mild challenge, we saw a reliable difference in the electrical activity of the heart,' says John Furedy, Ph.D., head of the laboratory where the study was run.

"The change was in the amplitude of the heart's T wave. This 'wave' occurs when the heart is pumping and pulling new blood in. The change indicated that, in less fit people, the heart overreacted to 'fight or flight' biochemicals, such as adrenalin, that are produced during psychological stress."[9]

Mental Benefits of Exercise

1. It enhances your mental abilities.

Exercise enhances one's mental abilities. In a series of tests, researchers at Scripps College in Claremont, California, compared sixty-two highly active people aged fifty-five to ninety-one with an equal number of non-exercisers of the same age. The one-and- one-half hour sessions of tests assessed reasoning, reaction time, and memory. The researchers found the high-exercise group performed significantly better in all reasoning tests, in all reaction-time tests, and in two of the three memory tests.[10]

2. It enhances your creative flow.

Creative flow is another benefit of exercise. Many people, myself included, find that the rhythmic flow of an exercise enhances the creative flow of ideas, also. I often spend time reflecting with the Lord while I exercise, and immediately afterward I sit down at my computer and download several outstanding ideas which the Lord has given to me during my prayer time. Try it — you might be amazed.

Why does exercise heal?

1. Exercise enhances the immune system.

From our earlier chapter on the lymph system, you already know one reason why this is true. Strenuous exercise speeds up the movement of lymph (our inner artillery) through the lymph system fifteen- to thirty-fold! So as you flex your body during exercise, you move your inner army of germ fighters into high gear. This is one of the most astounding insights I personally received from my study on health and nutrition.

2. Exercise reduces fat.

Those who exercise become leaner. Cancer thrives more readily in fatty tissue than lean tissue.

3. Exercise reduces constipation.

Constipation has been linked with colon cancer, and inactive people are more likely to be constipated. Exercise stimulates the peristaltic action of the intestines, and that results in regular and more frequent bowel movements.

4. Exercise increases blood flow.

Small arteries can begin to shut down through lack of physical activity. Exercise expands and re-opens these blood vessels. It is the flow of blood that oxygenates your body and carries away wastes. So exercise both detoxifies your system and oxygenates your cells.

What kinds of exercise should I do?

For years I assumed that doing aerobic exercise would be enough. However, I was missing two other categories of exercises which are also vitally important. A well-rounded fitness program **should incorporate** three basic components: 1) cardiovascular endurance, 2) muscular strength, and 3) flexibility. Following this guideline, any program you select should include exercises that increase heart and lung capacity, stretch tight muscle groups, and strengthen weak ones. Many people tend to neglect stretching exercises and end up with lower back pain. This is exactly what happened to me. So I have repented, and now follow a much more well-rounded exercise program.

Aerobic Exercise (three times a week)

Cardio-respiratory fitness refers to how well the lungs deliver oxygen to the blood and how well the heart and circulatory system send blood and its nutrients throughout the body. Programs that develop heart and lung capacity are often referred to as being aerobic, and they accomplish their goal by elevating the heart rate for a sustained period. Aerobic exercise typically serves as the foundation for any fitness program, since a healthy heart and lungs are essential to the safe and skillful performance of almost all activities and sports.

Depending upon your level of fitness and what you hope to achieve, most experts recommend a minimum of twenty minutes of aerobic exercise, three to five days a week. You may choose any activity that uses large muscle groups, that can be maintained continuously, and that is cardio-respiratory in nature. Examples include brisk walking, swimming, jogging, running, bicycling, cross-country skiing, skating, stair-climbing, hiking, dancing, basketball, soccer, and racque... or the speed of the workout, is crucial and is measured by how ... heart is made to beat. Usually the goal is to reach 65 to 90 percent or the exerciser's highest possible heart rate and sustain this rate for some length of time.

To determine your maximum safe heart rate, subtract your age from 220. During your exercise program you should not go over this rate. However, the target heart beat you want to sustain during aerobic exercise is 65 to 90 percent of your highest possible rate. So if you are forty, your target heart rate is between 117 and 162 (220 - 40 = 180. 180 X 65% = 117; 180 X 90% = 162).

Strength-building exercises (three times a week)

Muscular strength and endurance exercises use progressive resistance to increase the size and strength of muscle fibers, resulting in a greater physical ability to perform work. Weight- lifting machines, such as the Nautilus, are typical of the types of resistance equipment used in building strength. Push-ups, chin-ups, and curls produce similar results but require no special equipment. Strength-building is also an effective way of improving general fitness, converting fat to muscle, and increasing metabolic rate.

Stretching Exercises (once or twice daily)

Flexibility training is an aspect of fitness that is often neglected. However, 40 percent of your body is muscle, including some 650 voluntary muscles (muscles over which you have control). The goal of flexibility training is to increase the range of motion around a joint. As muscles become stronger through exercise, they also become tighter unless flexibility training is done.

Use slow, sustained stretches rather that bouncing, as bouncing can create microscopic tears in your muscles which will scar over as they heal and further diminish your flexibility. Since your muscles are more limber after you have exercised, it is recommended that you save your stretching until the close of your exercise period. That is different than I had been taught in the past, but I tried it and found that my muscles were much more relaxed after exercising, and they did stretch further and easier, with less strain. For a warm up, simply do your regular exercise at a slower pace for the first few minutes.

One awesome stretching exercise which really helped my lower back was the Ear-Knee-Stretch.[11] Sit on a chair and put your feet flat on the floor, with knees spread wide apart and hands on ankles. Let your torso sink between your knees to loosen your back a bit. Then slowly bend your torso to the right, until your right ear touches your right knee. Rotate your head slowly to the right. Raise your left arm until it is just short of hanging over your head. Hold for ten seconds, then slowly raise and repeat on the opposite side. Only one to three repetitions need to be done. I feel everything stretch from my legs right up through my back and to my neck. It is wonderful.

It is wise to vary your exercises so you are constantly working on a variety of muscles. This will also keep you from getting bored.

Getting a trainer

Some people enjoy going to an athletic club. Some of you may want to start a club in your church. Others prefer the privacy of their own homes. If you need assistance in how to do various exercises and how many should be done, any secular bookstore will carry several books on exercise, with pictures showing each. Go and browse and have a good time. After browsing for awhile myself, I picked up a book called *Your Personal Trainer* by Ann Goodsell, published by Better Homes and Gardens. One of Ann Goodsell's more famous clients is Olympic Gold Medalist Sally Gunnell. It was extremely helpful.

How Much Exercise Should I Do?

If you have not been exercising, START SLOWLY. Give your body a chance to adapt over the first few weeks. It will do so rapidly. If you have a major health problem, check with your doctor first. Even if you don't think you have a major health problem, it is advisable to check with a doctor before you begin an exercise program. Why take a chance? It is not necessary.

Twenty to thirty minutes a day, three to five days a week is sufficient to provide you with the health benefits mentioned in this chapter.

Moderate exercise will be fine. You do not need to kill yourself when you exercise. Enjoying yourself is much more important because then you will continue for months to come.

Finding time to exercise

How do you justify spending twenty to thirty minutes, three to five days a week on bodily exercise when you have so many other things you could and should be doing? There are several possibilities. One is to realize that for every hour you spend exercising, you gain an hour of life. Secondly, I find I am much more alert and effective for many hours after I have exercised, so I actually get much more done in much less time. Third, you can get many creative ideas when you are exercising, which when implemented, make you much more effective, with much less work. Fourth, you can use your exercise time for your devotional time also. You can pray or worship. You can use headphones and listen to praise and worship songs, or you can listen to the Bible on cassette, or you may want to intersperse this with teaching cassettes, motivational cassettes, etc.

If you walk for exercise, you can walk with your spouse or children or a close friend, and utilize the time building the relationship. Many spouses struggle to find time to talk together. Wouldn't it be fun to walk and talk together as a family?

Personally, I am always doing something else while I exercise, and my day is much more productive because of exercising in the morning.

Walking

Prevention magazine began a walking club in 1986 with more than 100,000 people. In 1992, they published a wonderfully motivational and instructional book entitled *Walking for Health*. If you are having trouble getting started exercising, read this book. It may be the motivation you need.

There are half-a-million regular mallwalkers in the United States. Mary, a lady from our church, met Jim as she walked in McKinley Mall in Hamburg, N.Y. A relationship budded, and soon our pastor conducted a mall wedding, sponsored by the owners of the mall. They also paid for their honeymoon. Not bad! Their story is included in the book published by Prevention.[12]

What exercise is best for you?

Do what you enjoy! Mile for mile, jogging burns only about 20 percent more calories than brisk walking, says James M. Rippe, M.D., Associate Professor of Medicine at the University of Massachusetts Medical Center in Worcester. Jogging jars your body with triple your body's weight every time you impact the ground, increasing the possibility of joint injury. When I jog, I try to stay on the grass or on a cushioned treadmill, under which I have put several layers of carpet.

My research for this chapter caused me to try something I never thought I would enjoy: walking. You see, I have been so in love with jogging for twenty-five years (because it stimulates those endorphins and I get a runners high) that I just felt nothing else could provide the same benefits. But when I discovered that walking was 80 percent as effective as jogging, and since my back had been giving me some problems, I tried walking on my treadmill. I was pleasantly surprised. I found I was walking at 4.5 miles an hour, which was only a bit slower than I jogged, which was at 5.2 miles an hour. I still worked up a sweat, and I still felt those endorphins jumping up and down in my body in excitement saying, "We're here! We're here!" I would usually jog 1.5 miles per day and do it in eighteen minutes. I found I could walk 1.5 miles in just twenty minutes. So the exercise time was only slightly increased, the results were the same and the jarring on my body was reduced by one-third. Perhaps I shouldn't have been so stubborn through the years. Perhaps I should have tried walking ten years ago when I first heard about it. Oh well, even though I strive to be a "learner", I still have emotional blocks that slow me down from time to time. Lord, heal my emotional and mental prejudices, so I can be a seeker of truth who walks in the light!

Handling common difficulties

1. Sore muscles

Sore muscles come from the build-up of lactic acid in your muscles as you exercise. This occurs because your body burns off both fat and muscle cells as you burn off calories. When it burns off muscle cells, you get lactic acid and soreness. One wonderful new discovery I have begun using is the Access fat conversion activity bar developed by Lawrence C. H. Wang, Ph.D. Professor of Animal and Human Physiology, University of Alberta in Edmonton. Dr. Wang discovered that adenosine, a chemical by-product of activity, blocks access to fat stores. Dr. Wang identified a natural substance that inhibits adenosine, enabling faster fat utilization and more powerful muscle strength for longer periods during exercise. I use it and have more energy while I exercise, and no soreness, even when doing exceptionally strenuous activities. It has really amazed me.

2. Blisters

Blisters can be avoided by starting slow, wearing an extra pair of socks, having comfortable shoes, and dry feet. If blisters strike, it is best to protect them, and let the fluid be re-absorbed into the body. You can get a pre-cut, doughnut-shaped bandage at your drugstore to surround the blistered area with a cushioned surface.

What does the Bible say about exercise?

The Bible does not say much about physical exercise. As a matter of fact, I can think of only one verse:

> "For [bodily exercise] profiteth little: but godliness is profitable unto all things, having promise of the life that now is, and of that which is to come" (I Timothy 4:8).

In this verse, Paul is comparing physical exercise to spiritual exercise. Obviously, since physical exercise is only for the life that now is, and spiritual exercise is for both the life that now is, and the life that is to come, spiritual exercise is far more important than physical exercise.

So if you can only do one, either physical or spiritual exercises, then do the spiritual ones. However, if you can couple the two together, as I suggested in this chapter, by praying and/or listening to Scripture on cassette, and getting creative flow from Almighty as you exercise, then perhaps you can do both. Or, perhaps you can find an extra thirty minutes when you watch TV or overeat on snacks, and use that time for exercise.

Even though bodily exercise is only for this life, this life could last eighty years. And to be healthy and vibrant during these eighty years, and to perhaps extend them to one hundred, will bring glory to God, since He has established a covenant of health with us.

> "Do you not know that your body is a temple of the Holy Spirit, who is in you, whom you have received from God? You are not your own; you have been bought with a price. Therefore honor God with your body" (I Cor. 6:20).

And finally, we need to take into account the context in which Paul wrote 1 Timothy 4:8. He was talking to people who did not have cars, who walked everywhere they went, who did not have automated equipment, but worked hard physically all day long. That group of people were **already doing** at least the moderate level of exercise which we have recommended in this chapter.

So, all in all, I think it brings glory to my God to do a moderate amount of exercise. It saves me 50 percent on my doctor's bills, so I now have money to invest other places, and it helps keep me alive, so I don't leave my wife as a widow, or our children as orphans.

Activities

1. Browse in a secular bookstore and pick up a good book on exercises. Examine it, so you get a feel for various exercises you could do in each of the three basic exercise categories.

2. Try a few exercises. Discuss with your spouse, or a friend, what exercises could be done together that would be fun for the two of you or for the whole family. Try them. See how they go.

3. Complete an exercise goals worksheet on the following page. Spend time in prayer and ask God what He wants you to do concerning exercise. Record what you are sensing in your spirit.

Additional Resources

Walking For Health, by Mark Bricklin and Maggie Spilner (Editors of <u>Prevention</u> magazine) This is an outstanding book which will motivate you to exercise and probably to begin walking for your health. If you need motivation to get started, get this book.

Family Guide to Natural Medicine, by Reader's Digest. Offers a good introduction to a wide variety of natural health practices, including exercise. Very well done, full color pictures throughout. It has some natural health practices which you may not agree with and may want to pass up.

Your Personal Trainer, by Ann Goodsell. An excellent book, teaching you how to do many exercises in all three exercise categories. It has pointers and full-color pictures throughout. If you are learning about exercise, you will greatly appreciate the features this book offers to beginners.

A. Record amounts and types of exercise:

Category   List Specific Activities and Length of Time

aerobic _____

_____

stretching_____

_____

muscle building_____

_____

B. Location(s) of exercises

_____

C. Expected benefits

physically _____

_____

_____

_____

emotionally _____

_____

_____

mentally_____

_____

_____

Beginning date _____

References

[1] "Exercise: A Little Helps a Lot," Consumer Reports on Health, volume 6, number 8 (August 1994), 89.

[2] *Eat Better, Live Better*, ed. Joseph Gardner (Pleasantville, NY: Reader's Digest, 1982), p. 320.

[3] *Walking for Health*, ed. Mark Bricklin and Maggie Spilner (Emmaus, PA: Rodale Press, 1992), p. 80.

[4] *Walking for Health*, p. 4.

[5] *Walking for Health*, p. 5.

[6] *Walking for Health*, p. 11.

[7] *Walking for Health*, p. 13.

[8] *Walking for Health*, p. 18.

[9] *Walking for Health*, pp. 80-81.

[10] *Walking for Health*, p. 4.

[11] *Walking for Health*, p. 175.

[12] *Walking for Health*, p. 102.

Chapter 10

The Healing Value of Faith, Hope and Love

Empowering For the Soul

God lists three things as abiding realities:

"But now abide faith, hope, love, these three; but the greatest of these is love" (1 Cor. 13:13 NASB).

God declares that the health of one's body is connected to the health of the soul, therefore providing the basis for psychosomatic (mind/body) relationships:

"Beloved, I pray that in all respects you may prosper and be in good health, just as your soul prospers" (3 John 2 NASB).

Norman Cousins made a big hit in 1979 with his book *Anatomy of an Illness*. In it he describes his own remarkable healing from terminal illness by laughing himself back to health. The truth is that laughter heals. It is medicine to our spirits, as well as our bodies.

"A merry heart maketh a cheerful countenance: but by sorrow of the heart the spirit is broken" (Proverbs 15:13).

"...he that is of a merry heart hath a continual feast" (Proverbs 15:15).

"A merry heart doeth good like a medicine: but a broken spirit drieth the bones" (Proverbs 17:22).

Now that I am over 40, I can feel the effects of harboring unforgiveness in my soul. The joints in my knees begin to ache. As soon as I forgive, the ache goes away. I find it amazing to see such a close correlation between my emotional state and my health. It is not that emotional states are wrong. Even the Bible says, "Be angry." However, the rest of that verse goes on to say, "yet do not sin; do not let the sun go down on your anger" (Eph. 4:26 NASB). Anger is not the problem. The problem is not processing my anger **that day**. It is when I harbor anger day after day that it becomes destructive to my system. The emotions I am supposed to live in, which provide health and life, are faith, hope, and love (1 Cor. 13:13). And this is not faith in the power of satan to rule and devastate this world, because the Bible is quite clear to say that "The Most High is ruler over the realm of mankind..." (Dan. 4:17).

Establish Inner Peace Through Proper Meditation Procedures

"Be anxious for nothing, but in everything by prayer and supplication with thanksgiving let your requests be made known to God, and the peace of God which surpasses all comprehension, shall guard your hearts and your minds in Christ Jesus. Finally, brethren, whatever is true, whatever is honorable, whatever is right, whatever is pure, whatever is lovely, whatever is of good repute, if there is any excellence and if anything worthy of praise, let your mind dwell on these things" (Phil. 4:6-8 NASB).

So the Bible recommends no anxiety but peace, instead. We are to maintain a positive emotional state by pondering positive things, things which are honorable and right, good and lovely. It is so easy to forget this injunction, to begin meditating on the corruption in government or the corruption in the medical society or the corruption in churches, and to move into anger, frustration, despair, cynicism and aggression.

The Bible says we should get together and find ways to stimulate one another to love and good deeds (Heb. 10:24,25). We are not to come together to discuss negative scenarios and how bad things are getting, and quote the latest crime, rape, and AIDS statistics. We are to gather to "stimulate one another to love and good deeds."

I wonder if God understood the health and medical implications of what He was commanding in the Holy Scriptures? I imagine that since He was our Creator and is our Sustainer, He is probably fully aware of the human body's biological responses to both anger and love. However, I was not, and so it was interesting to me to learn what modern science has discovered. The bottom line of their research is that anger kills and love heals. This has very important implications for me if I want to live many years in health and vitality. Let's take some time and explore what their research is showing.

The Brain/Emotion/Chemical Connection Within Our Bodies

Candace Pert, Ph.D., a visiting professor at the Center for Molecular and Behavioral Neuroscience at Rutgers University in Newark, New Jersey, states, "Our research shows that emotions are intimately connected with the entire physiology of the body....The chemical processes that mediate emotion occur not only within our brains, but also at many sites throughout the body — in fact on the very surfaces of every single cell."[1]

Endorphins, natural painkillers created in the body, do not just stay in the brain. Endorphins are processed in opiate receptors. These have traditionally been known to operate in the brain. However, recently opiate receptors have also been discovered in the immune system, in the lymph nodes, thymus gland, spleen, bone marrow and immune cells. Therefore, it is now clear from a biological perspective that the immune system is connected to the nervous system, involving the brain in the control of the disease-fighting process.

This helps me understand on a biological level what is happening when I confess, "By His stripes I am healed" (Isa. 53:5). ONE thing that is happening is that my brain, which in this case has been renewed with the Holy Scriptures, is telling every single cell in my body to be healed and instructing my immune system to enhance its disease-fighting capabilities. **I am not suggesting that this is all that is happening.** I believe there are very real spiritual forces, such as the anointing of the Holy Spirit, at work also, overcoming the power of sickness and disease. God causes ALL things to work together for good (Rom. 8:28).

This leads me to believe that in order to be healed, I want the renewing of my mind working together with the Word of God, the confession of the Word of God by my lips, and the flow of the anointing of the Holy Spirit. Lacking any of these important elements may hinder a full release of God's healing provision in our lives.

Short-term stress has been determined to bolster some aspects of immune function. However, **chronic stress** may cause the immune system to falter and health problems to arise. "When researchers from the University of California - Los Angeles recently examined the relationship between stressful life events and the development of col-orectal cancer in more than 1,000 men, for example, they found that those with a history of severe work-related problems were five times more likely to get colorectal cancer than men without job difficulties."[2] The colon is particularly sensitive to stress. "The same neuropeptides that are found in your brain and are associated with various emotional states also innervate every sphincter of your digestive system."[3]

A Sense of Helplessness

It is not just stress that deteriorates the immune system. Inappropriate responses to stress put us at risk of depressed immunity and possible disease. Rats who have no control over intermittent electrical shocks develop tumors faster than those who have access to a turn-off switch.

I have a turn-off switch to my stressful thoughts: hearing what God is saying to me about the situation. When I take my stress or anger to Him in prayer and He speaks back into my heart, I am healed and warmed, and my stress dissipates. I am sure most Christians have experienced this over and over. The sense of control that the Christian has is an awareness that **God** is in control of his life, and that his life is moving forward with purpose and meaning.

Anger Kills

Hostility is harmful to your health. There is some evidence to show that Type A personalities move more easily toward anger and hostility than do Type B personalities. Type A is the more aggressive personality style. They are the people who sit on the front edge of their chairs, ready to spring into action. They are always on the move, doing things; competitive; easily irritated by delays, having a low tolerance for frustration. Hard-hitting and ambitious, they are highly aggressive and easily angered. They cannot relax without feeling guilty, and have a tendency to finish other people's sentences. Type A people easily become impatient and demanding. They are quick to judge and quick to anger. I am Type A person myself. By "abiding in Jesus" I can overcome the potentially negative aspects of the Type A personality and not live in anger, hostility and stress.

Type B people are more laid-back. They sit all the way back in their chairs. They enjoy the experience of life more. They can enjoy "being" and do not have to be "doing" as much as the type A person does. They can switch off, play, and relax. Patti, my wife, is Type B.

In interviews with 142 patients scheduled for coronary angiography, it was found that equal proportions were Type A and B, possibly because all Americans eat a high-fat, high-cholesterol, low-fiber diet.

However, among those with moderately severe blockages, more than 70 percent were Type A; and among those with very severe blockages — at least two coronary arteries totally blocked off by arteriosclerotic plaques — more than 90 percent were Type A. Type A behavior is a real coronary disease risk factor.[4]

Eighteen hundred middle-aged men working at a Western Electric factory in Chicago were given an anger profile. It was found that those who at age twenty-five had scores in the upper half of the profile were four to five times more likely than those with lower scores to develop coronary disease and nearly seven times more likely to die from any cause.[5]

Caring Relationships

Stressed and hostile people tend to have fewer warm, caring relationships. This lack damages their health. In one study of 1300 heart patients who had returned home from the hospital, it was discovered that of those who were married or who had a confidant or both, only 17 percent were dead five years later. Of those who had neither a spouse nor a close confidant, 50 percent were dead. Giving and receiving love is essential for good health.[6]

Hostility also increases blood cholesterol levels and weakens the immune system.[7]

> "But now you also, put them all aside: anger, wrath, malice, slander, and abusive speech from your mouth" (Col. 3:8).

Hostility is characterized by cynicism, anger, and aggression. Therefore, I need to keep careful watch on the development of these emotions within my heart. They are the opposite of faith, hope, and love: the emotions which are to abide within me forever. Communing with Jesus purifies my emotions. As David took his emotions to the Lord in prayer in the Psalms, so I, too, take my emotions to God in prayer through journaling, and I find the same healing response as David did.

My Story

I discovered these truths about Type A personality behavior and high cholesterol the same week I had my cholesterol re-tested to see how I was doing. This is about six months after the testing and numbers I quoted you in the first chapter, where my cholesterol had fallen sixty-five points from 274 to 209 in ninety days. I had been exercising, eating mostly the Genesis diet, eating a cereal called Fiber One, taking

Cholestrex capsules from the health food store, and drinking Shak-lee's Heart Plan Formula. I was ecstatic about the drop in my cholesterol and continued with the exercise and Genesis diet. However, I quit the Cholestrex, Fiber One and Heart Plan Formula.

I was devastated to discover that my cholesterol had climbed back up to 253! It had gone up forty-four points, and was now only twenty-one points lower than when I had begun! So much for exercise and eating right. My first response was — Throw this book away — it doesn't work! (By the way, that is more a Type A response than a Type B!)

As I began to ponder the situation, the Lord reminded me of something that has been true so often in my life: The week before I am going to teach a particular truth, God often has me live through it, so it is very fresh in my heart and mind, and the truth is deepened within me.

I believe that is exactly what God is doing with me as I write this chapter. I "knew" that I was to live in faith, hope, and love and steer clear of stress, anger, and hostility. And I felt I was doing a pretty good job at it. However, in the book *Anger Kills*, Dr. Redford Williams lists forty-six questions which are part of a hostility profile. Dr. Williams contends that it is the hostility in the Type A personality which is the problem. If we can identify the hostility and remove it, we can lower cholesterol. I took the test, which measures the three underlying building-blocks which together create hostility: cynicism, anger, and aggression. According to his scoring key, I ranked high or very high in anger and aggression, with a total hostility score **in the range which causes health risk!**

Obviously, the test was flawed! I am a Spirit-filled believer who has written a book on *Communion With God* and another on *Abiding in Christ*. What does Dr. Williams know? On the other hand, **what was driving up my cholesterol?** I didn't even want to examine the possibilities because if I were to discover that I was less spiritual than I desired to be, I am not sure I could handle it. Tough on the old ego, you know. So I started where any good, self-protecting individual would. I re-read the section of Dr. Williams' book which explained why hostility increased cholesterol. Perhaps his reasoning was flawed. Here is what he said:

> "We have also found that this increased physiologic reactivity to stress is present among high Ho subjects [the Ho profile is a hostility profile] not only when they are being harassed in our lab but also when they are going about their normal daily activities. Consequently, men with high Ho scores show a larger increase of adrenalin

in their urine from overnight to daytime than do those with low Ho scores. Paralleling the correlation between anger and physiologic reactivity in the lab studies, the increase in adrenalin excretion was most pronounced in those hostile men who reported increased irritation levels during the day-time.

"Another very recent finding from our research into biologic mechanisms of hostility suggests that hostility can **magnify** the impact of another important risk factor, blood cholesterol, thereby making a high cholesterol level even worse for a hostile person. Among middle-aged men with high Ho scores, those with higher blood cholesterol levels secreted more adrenalin while performing mental tasks than did those with lower blood cholesterol levels."[8]

"Hostile men with high cholesterol, then, are more likely to have larger adrenalin responses to stress — a combination that compounds the likelihood of arteriosclerotic plaque build-up in their coronary arteries."[9]

"Several known effects of adrenalin...are probably responsible for their arteriosclerosis-promoting effects. First, they cause the blood pressure to rise and the heart to beat more rapidly, and both of these effects could increase risk of damage to the delicate inner lining of the arteries. Second, these stress hormones **cause fat cells to release fat into the bloodstream; if this fat is not burned up in the course of intense physical exercise, it is converted by the liver into cholesterol, thereby making more cholesterol available in the blood for incorporation into arteriosclerotic plaques.** And third, adrenalin...cause[s] the platelets circulating in the blood to become much more 'sticky', thereby stimulating them to stick to damaged areas on the artery lining, where they clump and release other chemicals that are believed to stimulate the growth of arteriosclerotic plaques."[10]

Incidentally, Dr. Williams mentions that he found that low-hostility women on birth control pills were just as hyperactive to harassment as high-hostility men. So being on contraceptives may cancel out some of the protection enjoyed by non-hostile women.

I had not fully grasped the fact that only a portion of our blood cholesterol comes from the food we eat and the rest is produced by our livers.[11] I went back to the book *The McDougall Plan* and reviewed what he had said about cholesterol. Often I find I don't **see** something until I have first lived it. Here is what McDougall says: "The body produces between 500 and 1000 milligrams of cholesterol per day, which is enough to supply our needs. When we eat the diet commonly consumed by people of affluent societies, we take in an additional 500 to 1000

milligrams a day...."[12] If I am living with stress, the amount of cholesterol produced by my body is elevated considerably. I thus offset the
benefits of my low-cholesterol diet because stress over-stimulates my
liver to produce excess cholesterol.

After reviewing Dr. Williams' reasoning, I was convinced that living
under stress or with hostility did trigger high cholesterol. It even made
me realize that my exercise program should be non-stress-producing
and non-competitive, or I could find myself producing more cholesterol
while I exercised, rather than decreasing it.

Next, I went back to the forty-six questions on the hostility questionnaire to see which ones made my score high. Here is some of what I
found: I ranked higher in cynicism because I do not believe politicians
are trustworthy, and I do not believe that if you put people on the honor
system, they wouldn't sneak in to see a movie without paying because
they know that to do so would be wrong.

The questionnaire said that my anger and aggression were evidenced
by becoming stressed by such things as teen-agers driving by with the
car stereo blaring acid rock; wanting to put away every drug pusher,
rather than seek out ways to reach and change them; feeling AIDS is
usually a result of irresponsible behavior rather than seeing it as a major
tragedy; becoming irritated and annoyed when stuck in a traffic jam,
rather than simply staying relaxed; feeling annoyed when another
driver cuts ahead of me in traffic, rather than simply staying further
back behind him; wanting to correct people with ignorant beliefs rather
than letting it pass; butting in to help a slow speaker finish his sentence,
rather than listening until he finishes; wanting to lash out at terrorists
who attack others, rather than wondering how people can be so cruel.

So my un-redeemed nature may be tempted to blow up abortion
clinics! I always considered that righteous indignation, not hostility or
aggression. What do you think? If the above things demonstrate cynicism, anger, aggression, and hostility, then there is a lot of hostility in
the Christian community to which I minister. I (we) never considered
it wrong. I just felt that was the way any good Bible-believing fervent
Christian was to respond.

So I checked with my wife to see if a Type B personality would really
answer the questions differently than I did. Of course, you do realize
that my perspective on life IS RIGHT AND BALANCED AND
BIBLICAL! AND I CAN PROVE IT FROM SCRIPTURE! I have
even been trying to get Patti to change so, she could become more like

me. Well, sure enough, her answers were opposite, **and she has low cholesterol and mine is high**.

Now, this is hard to take. It is clear that my body is not working properly. My cholesterol is way too high, and my diet is not causing it, nor is lack of exercise. The only thing that can be causing it is my intense inner drive ("hostility" is the negative word for it). Well, I guess it is time for a reality check. Obviously, there is something about living in faith, hope, love, peace, and joy which I have not yet internalized into my personality structure. And if I don't, I will probably die ten to twenty years earlier than God intended. I guess I will just have to go back to the school of the Holy Spirit, and learn some new inner ways of living and responding to life.

And in the meantime, while I am learning, I am going back on Fiber One and Cholestrex and possibly even Shak-lee's Heart Plan Formula. I will experiment a bit with these different products and have my cholesterol checked every two months to find which one or combination of the above is required to get and keep my cholesterol down. I do believe that genetics comes into play, and some people's systems do produce more cholesterol. These people will have a greater struggle to keep it down, even when doing all the right things.

And guess what my wife began doing as soon as we made this discovery. The very next day she got out the recipe book that came with her electric breadmaker, and began making me homemade bread which was high in water-soluble fibers, and thus designed to lower cholesterol. Now throughout the day I can munch on some bread that will help lower my cholesterol. Thanks, Patti! Incidentally, in the colon, fiber transforms into substances that interfere with the body's production of cholesterol.

I hope this story helps some of you Type A people who are reading. You may want to purchase the book *Anger Kills*, just so you can take the hostility test. (Plus, it lists seventeen strategies for controlling hostility). Another good book to purchase is *Adrenalin & Stress* by Dr. Archibald D. Hart.

At least I am beginning to get answers concerning my cholesterol, and beginning to understand where I need to put my efforts. And do you know what? Once I have succeeded in mastering my cholesterol levels, I will have gained personality traits which will make me a much more effective person in life. I suspect that I am living too intensely, too impatiently. I push too hard, both myself and others. I strive more than necessary. I need to learn to "kick back" more, at least in my inner attitudinal poise. I need to live in the revelation that God's Spirit can accomplish more in a moment than I ever can in a month, and that when I relax internally, I am more open to His wonderful creative flow. I will get just as much done, probably even much more, if I stay relaxed and tuned to His Holy Spirit.

Incidentally, some people do not express their hostility and aggression outwardly. Some people turn it inward and it attacks their bodies in other ways. Stress internalized produces many gastronomical problems.

Emotions must be effectively processed at the root level each time they occur. That is the only effective solution.

How to Process Emotions Quickly and Effectively

Dr. Redford Williams offers seventeen strategies for controlling hostility in his book *Anger Kills*. They comprise seventeen chapters of his book and include the following: reason with yourself; stop hostile thoughts, feelings, and urges; distract yourself; meditate; avoid over-stimulation; assert yourself; care for a pet; listen; practice trusting others; take on community service; increase your empathy; be tolerant; forgive; have a confidant; laugh at yourself; become more religious; pretend today is your last.

You might want to go back over that list, reading slowly, pondering and praying about it. Some of those titles may spark insight and direction within you. Or you just might want to purchase the book and use it in your devotional time for a month or so.

When I look at the Bible, I see David processing his emotions before the Lord in prayer using music and writing. He wrote a psalm (which means "to be sung") expressing his inner intensity, followed by a quiet time of listening for what the Lord would speak back. He then wrote down what the Lord said. He closed with praise and worship. A good example of this is Psalm 61. In verse one, he says that his heart is faint, and in the first four verses he is asking God to meet him. At the end of verse four he has a "Selah" time, which means "pause, crescendo or musical interlude" (see marginal reference of New American Standard Bible). Step one, therefore, is to write and/or sing your problem to God. Step two is to listen in your heart for God to speak back. Have music in the background to attune your soul to God. Step three is in verses 5 through 7, where he writes down what he believes God is saying during the "Selah" time. The final step is found in verse eight: David sings praise to God for what He has said to him.

This kind of praying involves several things which may not be found in our twentieth century prayer times. It involves singing, writing, listening, hearing back the still small voice of God within, speaking and singing forth what God was saying, and then closing with praise for what God has said. I do teach this process in other books. I also have a brief appendix in this book on hearing God's voice. I believe that to receive the maximum healing God wants to give us through prayer, we need to incorporate some of these wonderful steps which David took in the Psalms. They are obviously there for our instruction, so we can learn (1 Cor. 10:11).

An example of journaling (modern psalm writing) between God and Mark Virkler.

Lord, what would you want to say to us about our emotions and our mind?

"Mark, you choose the emotions which will dominate your life. Yes, there are many emotions which push to the surface and seek to be heard and entertained; however, you have the power of choice as to which one you will allow to flood your being. If you choose fear, you will be defeated. If you choose faith, you will overcome. Think not that there is anything ethereal about this. This is the essence of life. Communing with Me and faith are the essence of life, because I am the essence of life. When one experiences Me, he is full of faith. When one experiences fear he is full of the evil one. Think not that this is strange. This is the essence of life. Everyone experiences this every day. Everyone knows in his spirit that this is true. Only the mind would argue with the concepts. The heart already bears witness to the truth. So fear not to share this publicly in your book. It is of Me.

"Mark, concerning your emotions and your health: Positive emotions emit positive energies. Negative emotions emit negative energies. Faith, hope and love emit life forever. Anger, fear, and guilt result in death. Choose life. Choose freedom in Me. Choose life evermore and you will be whole.

"Am I so hard to come to that one would set Me aside? Am I so unreal as to not have tangible value in one's life? No! And again I say unto you, No! I am the Giver of Life. I am the Receiver of life. I am Life evermore. He who abides in Me abides in life. He who abides in himself abides in death. Come and live in Me that your joy may be full. Come enjoy full life. I am not far away. I am the life you live and the breath you breathe. I am the wind that blows where it wills, and no one knows where it comes from or where it goes. I am the Great I Am. I am the Lord of All. And yet, I am the Lover of your soul.

"I am the One who sent My Son to die for you on Calvary. I am the One who wept when we were separated in the Garden of Eden. I am the One who sent the second Adam. I am the One who restored all things. I love you, Mark, and I love each one reading these words. They are My chosen ones. They are the ones I gave my life for.

"Come to Me, My children, and I will make you whole. Come to Me, My children, and I will make you whole. Come to Me, My children, and I will make you whole. You must only **come to Me.** Will you do that?"

Lord, I will come. Heal my soul, I pray. I come to You.

I learned to journal and dialogue with God, as in the above example, in 1979 when I learned how to hear God's voice. Patti and I have written four books about it: *Communion With God, Dialogue With God, Counseled by God Textbook,* and *Counseled by God Workbook.* (These can be studied individually or in a group.) There have been times in the past when I have journaled and worshiped and sung much more to God in the mornings than I am currently doing, and I felt much greater levels of inner peace than I do currently. I think in light of the current fruit of my life as revealed in this chapter (i.e. health-damaging cholesterol levels), I must go back to that once again. So I will.

It has been easy for me to say, "God made me this way" (intense) and find Scriptures to prove my approach is acceptable (Paul, Peter). Doing that, of course, **becomes a barrier** to keep me from changing. However, if we can test something by its fruit, the fruit of my belief system is high cholesterol, as well as many other negative dynamics. Since I value God's direction through life's experiences, I have decided to let my cholesterol level help lead me into the realization that I must live less intensely and even become a barometer of sorts, indicating when I have mastered these new skills.

You may want to pick up a Stress Monitor card which clearly reveals your level of tension within within seconds. Many locations carry them. (Also available using the order form at the end of this book.)

A group of executives who scored high on the stress scale were studied. One hundred who stayed healthy under stress and one hundred who became ill were chosen for study. It was found that the hundred who stayed healthy felt more committed, felt more in control and had bigger appetites for challenge (i.e. were more "hardy") than those who got sick. A test for "hardyness" can be found in the book *Your Emotions and Your Health*. By learning to enhance your hardyness, you can handle stress more effectively.

Enhancing Interpersonal Communication

Close, loving relationships are great enhancers of health. These do not come naturally, as most of us have discovered. We need to cultivate social skills, so that we can deepen friendships. We need to learn how to listen, and how to be assertive without hurting the other person. We need to know how to express love. Perhaps you have given these things some thought. Perhaps you have taken a course on such topics. Perhaps not. This is the stuff life and health is made of. We would surely do ourselves a favor to take a course or read a book or two in this area. Both Protestant and Catholic churches offer marriage enhancement seminars. I think every couple would benefit greatly by taking one.

Patti and I have chosen to. The Protestant version of the marriage encounter which Patti and I went to is called Nova Shalom. We have also gone for a week of counseling at Elijah House in Post Falls, Idaho with Mark Sanford. This was extremely valuable in helping us discover and heal inner judgments and inner vows which we had both made in our earlier lives, and which were still wreaking havoc in our lives because of the spiritual laws of sowing and reaping and the hundredfold return. We have also found extreme benefit in going through the video series together, "Love is a Decision" by Gary Smalley.

My brother, Dr. Henry Virkler, has written an outstanding book entitled *Speaking Your Mind Without Stepping on Toes*. It can be used individually, as a couple, or in cell groups and will help one build relationship skills.

Patti and I have also begun working through a book entitled *Couple Communication I - Talking and Listening Together* by Sherod Miller, Phyllis Miller, Elam W. Nunnally, and Daniel B. Wackman. It is available from Interpersonal Communication Programs, Inc. 7201 South Broadway Littletown, Colo. 80122. (303) 794-1764.

The book *Adrenalin & Stress* offers a lot of insight on stress control and what stress and Type A behavior do to one's body. The author, Dr. Archibald D. Hart, is Dean of the Graduate School of Psychology and Professor of Psychology at Fuller Theological Seminary.

Recommended Reading

Anger Kills by Redford Williams, M.D.

Speaking Your Mind Without Stepping on Toes by Henry A. Virkler

None of These Diseases by S.I. McMillen, M.D.

Communion With God by Mark & Patti Virkler

Dialogue With God by Mark & Patti Virkler

Counseled by God Textbook by Mark and Patti Virkler

Counseled by God Workbook by Mark and Patti Virkler

Adrenalin & Stress by Dr. Archibald D. Hart

Everyday Health Tips - 2000 Practical Things for Better Health and Happiness by the editors of <u>Prevention</u> magazine.

References

[1] Stocker, Sharon, "Shelter Your Health from Emotional Stress," Prevention, volume 46 number 4 (April 1994), p. 74.

[2] Stocker, p. 76.

[3] Stocker, p. 77.

[4] Williams, Redford and Virginia Williams, *Anger Kills* (New York: Random House, 1993), p. 33.

[5] Williams, p. 37.

[6] Williams, p. 44.

[7] Williams, p. 50.

[8] Williams, p. 48.

[9] Williams, p. 49.

[10] Williams, p. 50.

[11] Hart, Archibald, *Adrenalin & Stress* (Waco, TX: Word, 1986), p. 100.

[12] McDougall, John, *TheMcDougall Plan*, p. 63.

Chapter 11

The Value of Spirit-Anointed Healing Prayer

Empowering For the Spirit

"God anointed Jesus of Nazareth with the Holy Ghost and with power: who went about doing good, ... healing all that were oppressed of the devil; for God was with Him" (Acts 10:38).

"Verily, verily, I say unto you, He that believeth on me, the works that I do shall he do also; and greater works than these shall he do; because I go unto my Father" (John 14:12).

"You shall receive power when the Holy Spirit has come upon you..." (Acts 1:8).

"And seizing him by the right hand, he [Peter] raised him up; and immediately his feet and his ankles were strengthened. And with a leap, he stood up-right and began to walk; and he entered the temple with them, walking and leaping and praising God" (Acts 3:7,8).

Our Bodies Are Programmed to Heal

God has programmed healing into every cell of our bodies, regardless of whether we are Christians or not. God has a passion to see us well, and He has made every provision for that eventuality. He has given us His laws, which if followed, will keep us well. And He has given us an anointing of the Holy Spirit Who can and will sovereignly intervene when we become sick, and overwhelm our bodies with health once again, so we have a new foundation of health and strength in our lives.

Whenever you cut your skin or burn or scrape your finger, your body goes on immediate alert and sends thousands of cells to the damaged area to heal it. Your cells never ask, "Is it God's will to heal in this situation?" There is no possibility that the cells would say, "Well, I guess we will just sit this one out to teach the person a lesson through this particular sickness." No, every cell continuously performs its healing function in your body. If it is given the tools it needs to work with, it will be effective in maintaining your body's health.

The evidence is clear to me that God's intention is that we be well. Scripture teaches it. Jesus' ministry demonstrates it. Every cell of our bodies reveals it on a moment-by-moment basis. Whenever we hurt ourselves, our instinctive reaction is to seek solutions to get better. Anything contrary to this is contrary to the way God has programmed our cells, our hearts, and our minds.

Divine Assistance of the Healing Process

One of God's covenants with His people is, "I am the Lord that healeth thee (literally, the Lord your health)" (Exodus 15:26). The prerequisites to receive His healing are:

1) Diligently hearken to the voice of the Lord thy God, and
2) Do that which is right in His sight, and
3) Give ear to His commandments, and
4) Keep all His statutes.

How is that for a list of prerequisites for health? This helps clarify in my mind why so many are sick.

Prerequisite # 1: Many do not believe God is speaking today. Of those who do believe He speaks, many do not know how to hear His voice. Many who do know how to hear His voice do not trust those inner impressions or follow them because we live in a culture which pressures us so much to worship rationalism, and discard inner impression.

Prerequisite # 2: Many do not do what is right, but are dishonest, greedy seekers of their own pleasure, their stomachs being their gods.

Prerequisite # 3: Many do not devote their lives to learning what the commandments of God are and how to effectively appropriate them in their lives.

Prerequisite # 4: For years I didn't even believe most of His statutes were for me. I thought that the Old Testament statutes were for the Israelites. The Gospels are a description of how Jesus lived, but not a way I could expect to live myself. I was taught that the book of Acts is a transitional book, and the commands and experiences contained therein do not directly relate to my life. Of course, the book of Revelation is for the future. So in my opinion, most of the statutes in the Bible did not even relate to me, even though I considered myself a Bible-believing Christian. I did believe the Bible. I just didn't believe most of it was for me. I am not sure that that put me very much ahead of the liberals (whom I scorned) who do not even believe the Bible is the Word of God. Incidentally, much of my growth as a Christian has been to realize that the entire Bible (all statutes and experiences) is to be lived by me today, unless, of course, Jesus in the New Testament specifically stated that He has fulfilled a particular statute in the Old Testament and has now modified it for me.

In summary, the children of God have been offered a special covenant of health with God and do not need to experience the same statistics of disease and death as the one who does not follow God's ways and His voice.

Jesus Healed ALL Who Came

Jesus healed continuously. He laid His hands on those who were brought to Him, spoke a word over them, and they were healed. Often, the casting out of demons accompanied His healing ministry. He never turned away a single person.

Following are copies of Appendices D and E of John Wimber's book *Power Healing*. They list forty-one examples of Jesus ministering healing, and twenty-eight examples of the disciples ministering healing. Anyone interested in either understanding or developing a healing ministry should read Wimber's book. It is one of the best.

An Overview of the Healing Ministry of Jesus

#	Description	Matthew	Mark	Luke	John
1.	Man with unclean spirit		1:23-25	4:33-35	
2.	Peter's mother-in-law	8:14,15	1:30,31	4:38,39	
3.	Multitudes	8:16,17	1:32-34	4:40,41	
4.	Many demons		1:39		
5.	Leper	8:2-4	1:40-42	5:12,13	
6.	Paralytic	9:2-7	2:3-5	5:17-25	

#	Description	Matthew	Mark	Luke	John
7.	Man with withered hand	12:9-13	3:1-5	6:6-10	
8.	Multitudes	12:15,16	3:10,11		
9.	Gadarene demoniac	8:28-32	5:1-13	8:26-33	
10.	Jairus's daughter	23-25	35-43	49-56	
11.	Women with issue of blood	9:20-22	5:25-34	8:43-48	
12.	A few sick people	13:58	6:5,6		
13.	Multitudes	14:34-36	6:55,56		
14.	Syro-phoenician's daughter	15:22-28	7:24-30		
15.	Deaf and dumb man		7:32-35		
16.	Blind man		8:22-26		
17.	Child with evil spirit	17:14-18	9:14-27	9:38-43	
18.	Blind Bartimaeus	20:30-34	10:46-52	18:35-43	
19.	Centurion's servant	8:5-13		7:2-10	
20.	Two blind men	9:27-30			
21.	Dumb demoniac	9:32-33			
22.	Blind and dumb demoniac	12:22		11:14	
23.	Multitudes	4:23		6:17-19	
24.	Multitudes	9:35			
25.	Multitudes	11:4,5		7:21	
26.	Multitudes	14:14		9:11	6:2
27.	Great multitudes	15:30			
28.	Great multitudes	19:2			
29.	Blind and lame in Temple	21:14			
30.	Widow's son			7:11-15	
31.	Mary Magdalene & others			8:2	
32.	Crippled woman			13:10-13	

#	Description	Matthew	Mark	Luke	John
33.	Man with dropsy			14:1-4	
34.	Ten lepers			17:11-19	
35.	Servant's ear			22:49-51	
36.	Multitudes			5:15	
37.	Various persons			13:32	
38.	Nobleman's son				4:46-53
39.	Invalid				5:2-9
40.	Man born blind				9:1-7
41.	Lazarus				11:1-44

The Healing Ministry of the Disciples

#	Description	Matthew	Mark	Luke	Acts
1.	Jesus' ministry described	11:2-6		7:18-23	
2.	The Twelve sent	10:1-11:1	3:13-19	9:1-11	
3.	The Seventy- two sent			10:1-24	
4.	Disciples attempt to cast out demons	17:14-21	9:14-29	9:37-45	
5.	Power to bind & loose	16:13-20			
6.	Great Commission	28:16-20	16:14-20	24:44-53	1:1-11
7.	Jesus' Ministry Described				2:22
8.	Signs & wonders at Apostles' hands				2:42-47
9.	Healing of lame beggar				3:1-4:22
10.	Prayer for confidence & healing signs				4:23-31
11.	Signs & wonders at Apostles' hands				5:12-16
12.	Ministry of Stephen				6:8-15
13.	Ministry of Philip				8:4-13
14.	Ananias and Saul				9:10-19

#	Description	Matthew	Mark	Luke	Acts
15.	Peter heals Aeneas (Lydda)				9:32-35
16.	Peter heals Dorcas (Joppa)				9:36-43
17.	The ministry of Jesus				10:34-41
18.	Magician Struck Blind by Paul				13:4-12
19.	Paul & Barnabas in Iconium				14:1-7
20.	Lame Man at Lystra				14:8-18
21.	Paul Raised at Lystra				14:19,20
22.	Slave Girl at Philippi				16:16-40
23.	Paul at Ephesus				19:8-20
24.	Eutychus Raised from the dead				20:7-12
25.	Paul recalls Ananias				22:12-21
26.	Paul on Malta				28:1-10
27.	Galatians 3:5				
28.	Hebrews 2:4				

There Are Various Levels of Healing Power

Simple touch

It appears to me that there are a variety of levels of healing power which can be tapped. First of all, touch is healing. Studies have been performed in hospitals showing that when nurses spend more time touching patients, the healing process is speeded up in their bodies.

Flow from man's spirit

Secondly, since man is made in the image of God, and man has a spirit, there is an energy in man's spirit which can be released when one ministers to another. Humanists have discovered and utilized this power, as have some New Age believers. Personally, I do not think we should seek to tap **our** spirits' power. Instead, we should unite our spirits with the Holy Spirit, which is what happens at the point of salvation. The one who joins himself to the Lord is one spirit with Him (1 Cor. 6:17). This moves us up to level three.

The believer's anointing

The third level is the anointing of the Holy Spirit, which is within the believer (1 John 2:27). This energizing work of the Holy Spirit **within** can be released through prayer and the laying on of hands. The intensity of this anointing's flow can be increased or decreased through either appropriate or in-appropriate actions. That is why the Bible cautions us not to "grieve the Holy Spirit of God, by Whom you were sealed for the day of redemption" (Eph. 4:30).

The anointing for ministry

The fourth level of healing power is the anointing of the Holy Spirit **upon** the believer. "You shall receive power when the Holy Spirit has come UPON you" (Acts 1:8). This is an even greater anointing (for ministry) than the anointing of the Holy Spirit **within** the believer. This anointing can be increased or decreased also.

The corporate anointing

The fifth level of healing power is the corporate anointing of the Holy Spirit upon a gathering of believers. For example, Jesus "did not many mighty works there because of their unbelief" (Matt. 13:58). So we see that the faith level of the corporate gathering (and perhaps, other things) can affect the release of the anointing to heal. This corporate anointing can be increased or decreased.

New Age Counterfeits in the Form of Spirit Guides

When I began this study on healing, a Christian wrote to me and shared his experience. As he explored diet, health, and healing he got mixed up with the New Age movement, so he backed away from the area rather confused. He was anxious to see how I made out. Well, contacting "spirit guides" is one important area where confusion can exist, and Christians can easily fall into error. The demonic counterpart to level four, the anointing for ministry, would be the use of "spirit guides" and familiar spirits. Use of spirit guides is strictly forbidden in the Bible (Deut. 18:10-13) and needs to be rejected by the Christian. (I would also steer clear of all paraphernalia that goes with this, including crystals, etc.) This counterfeit is practiced in the New Age movement and cult and occult groups.

The Spirit who guides the Christian is the Holy Spirit. My conviction as a Christian is that we are to live in fellowship with the Holy Spirit. The New Age practitioner or cultist walks in error as he precipitates healing power through other spirit guides. Even if the New Age believer's spirit guide appears very loving and kind, it is dangerous because the Bible says that satan can come as an "angel of light" (2 Cor. 11:14). The **only truly safe way into the realm of the Spirit** is for the committed Christian who has made Jesus his Lord and Savior and been washed in the blood of the Lamb, to experience fellowship with the Holy Spirit (2 Cor. 13:14) as he walks and ministers in the anointing of the Spirit (Gal. 5:18,25).

Two Extremes to Avoid

We should avoid two extremes. We should not fear moving in the power of the Holy Spirit simply because there is a counterfeit in satan's realm. Many Christians have thrown the baby out with the bath water. They are afraid of a lot of natural healing practices and call them **all** New Age. Although many people who follow many of the things in this book are New Age believers, and we, as Christians, do need to practice much wisdom and discernment, we also need to be **more careful not to reject** healthy habits because of **unhealthy** narrow-mindedness!

Nor should we allow ourselves to be deceived by getting involved with angels of light or spirit guides. Stay clear of anything that exalts SELF and the power within. The New Age also always refers to tapping into the universal energy and cosmic force rather than a **personal** God through Jesus Christ.

Defining the Anointing of the Holy Spirit WITHIN the Believer

This is the **most basic anointing** which the believer has. All other anointings are built upon this anointing.

> "But the **anointing** which ye have received of Him **abideth in you,** and ye need not that any man teach you: but as the same anointing teacheth you of all things, and is truth, and is no lie, and even as it hath taught you, ye shall abide in Him" (1 John 2:27).

"And the peace of God, which passeth all understanding, shall keep your hearts and minds through Christ Jesus" (Philippians 4:7).

"The Spirit Himself beareth witness with our spirit, that we are the children of God" (Romans 8:16).

What is this anointing **within** the believer? According to the above verses, it abides in the believer and teaches us from within. It can provide peace or unrest. It bears witness in our spirits. I think all Christians have sensed it. You may feel a check in your spirit or a release in your spirit. I suppose it can be confused with other checks in our hearts at times. That is why the "inner anointing" is only one of several ways that I hear God's voice in my life.

I use six primary pillars to determine God's leading in my life. One pillar is the inner anointing. A second, is illumined Scriptures which God brings to my heart and mind. A third pillar is the illumined counsel of other godly people; a fourth, is illumined anointed thoughts. The fifth, is an illumined understanding of the experiences of life, and the final, is direct revelation through God's voice or a divine flow of dream or vision. When God's voice is confirmed through all six pillars, I have a high level of confidence that I am seeing as much truth as I can see at this point in my life.

If I get an impression (which often is from the Lord), I test it against the inner anointing, or the peace, deep in my spirit. I say, "Lord Jesus Christ, is this impression from You?" If I feel "peace" in my spirit, then I move ahead. If I feel a check, then I wait. Once again, the programming of my own heart can interfere with the clear leading of the Holy Spirit, who is in union with my spirit. There are several things I do to get beyond my own heart, including: worshipping for awhile in the Lord's presence; fixing my eyes upon Jesus; lifting up my eyes to Him; praying in tongues for awhile; sleeping on it and seeing what my spirit's impressions are in the morning; prayerfully mulling over Scriptures; and asking for input from other spiritual counselors.

Defining the Anointing of the Holy Spirit UPON the Believer

This is the anointing for ministry (Acts 1:8). This is where there is a flow of divine power through you which overflows to others as you minister God to them. It flows out from you. It often saturates your clothing, and it can be sensed leaving your body. It appears to be some form of spiritual energy. As Jesus was ministering;

"a woman who had had a hemorrhage for twelve years, and had endured much at the hands of many physicians, and had spent all that she had and was not helped at all, but rather had grown worse, after hearing about Jesus came up in the crowd behind Him, and touched His cloak, for she thought, 'If I just touch His garments, I shall get well.' And immediately the flow of her blood was dried up; and she felt in her body that she was healed of her affliction. And immediately Jesus, perceiving in Himself that the power proceeding from Him had gone forth, turned around in the crowd and said, 'Who touched My garments?'" (Mark 5:25-30)

We can learn much about how the healing anointing can be experienced in our lives from just these few verses. 1) When medicine and doctors don't help, people often call out to God. 2) The woman's faith helped in releasing the healing anointing because many others were touching him and not being healed (vs. 31). 3) She had faith that a specific action would precipitate the healing anointing, and it did! 4) Jesus could sense the anointing being released from Him. 5) The healing anointing can saturate inanimate objects like Jesus' clothes. 6) Touch or contact is one good way to release the anointing (see also Luke 6:19). 7) The woman could feel the anointing entering her body and healing the affliction.

The last paragraph is worth pondering and praying over for awhile, as you ask yourself the question, "How and when have I experienced similar things?" It is as we learn to become sensitive to this inner flow and release of the power of God in and through us that we become effective channels of the healing anointing.

Three Words Describing the POWER of God

I want to do everything I can to understand this anointing power — how it is given, how it is sensed, and how it is released — because therein lies a healing miracle which can remove much pain and suffering and save people's lives. There are three key words in the New Testament translated "power".

Exousia

This word occurs about 108 times and its main meaning is "authority." God has given us the authority to heal the sick.

Dunamis

This word occurs about 118 times in the New Testament and is the root word of "dynamite". It means strength, force, ability, capacity, resources.

Energes

This word and its forms occur about 31 times in the New Testament, and it means "active energy...adapted to accomplish a thing." (Definition from the *Analytical Greek Lexicon* by Zondervan).

To release divine power through the healing anointing, one begins with the realization that God has granted him the authority to heal (*exousia*). He then cultivates the growth of divine power (*dunamis*) within his spirit. In healing prayer, he releases this active energy (*energes*), focusing the flow of divine power within him to perform healing in a person's body.

To master the release of divine healing power through you, you are asked to accomplish three different things:

First, you must become completely convinced, based on the authority of the Holy Scriptures, that God wants you to minister healing, and that He has given you the authority to heal and overcome all the works of the enemy.

Second, you must cultivate the expansion of the active power (*dunamis*) of the Holy Spirit within your spirit, soul and body.

Third, you must learn to release the Holy Spirit's energy (*energes*) through you to accomplish specific healing objectives.

These three steps require Bible knowledge and a growing sensitivity to the working of the Holy Spirit within you. Generally, God takes His leaders apart from life for awhile in order to learn this sensitivity. Joseph learned it (i.e. the ability to interpret dreams) in a prison. Moses learned it in the wilderness, as did Paul and Jesus. Notice the difference between Jesus going out to the wilderness and returning back from the wilderness: Luke 4:1 "Jesus, **full** of the Holy Spirit...was led into the wilderness." Luke 4:14 "...Jesus returned...in the **power** of the Spirit...." So His stay in the wilderness transformed Him from a "fullness" to a "power". His next action was to perform His first miracle at the wedding feast in Cana.

There is something we learn when we get alone and discern our hearts and spirits that increases within us the ability to release the power of God in a way that we were previously not able. This learning is not a classroom learning. It is not a book thing. It is a learning to become sensitive to sensations within our being — learning to sense the movements of God within us. The results?

> "And all the multitude were trying to touch Him, for power was coming from Him and healing them all" (Luke 6:19).

> "And the power of the Lord was present for Him to perform healing" (Luke 5:17).

> "From his innermost being shall flow rivers of living water...but this He spoke of the Spirit, whom those who believed in Him were to receive; for the Spirit was not yet given, because Jesus was not yet glorified" (John 7:38,39).

> "And God was performing extraordinary miracles by the hands of Paul, so that handkerchiefs or aprons were even carried from his body to the sick, and the diseases left them and the evil spirits went out" (Acts 19:11,12).

> "It is the Spirit who gives life..." (John 6:63).

> "Stay in the city until you are clothed with power from on high" (Luke 24:49).

The Teacher

He never taught a lesson in a classroom... He had no tools to work with, such as blackboards, maps or charts... He used no subject outlines, kept no records, gave no grades, and His only text was ancient and well-worn... His students were the poor, the lame, the deaf, the blind, the outcast — and His method was the same with all who came to hear and learn... He opened eyes with faith... He opened ears with simple truth... and opened hearts with love, a love born of forgiveness... A gentle man, a humble man, He asked and won no honors, no gold awards of tribute to His expertise or wisdom... And yet this quiet teacher from the hills of Galilee has fed the needs, fulfilled the hopes, and changed the lives of many millions... For what He taught brought heaven to earth and revealed God's heart to mankind (Author unknown).

What Does the Anointing Feel Like?

Mark 5:25-30 — You can feel energy leave you.

Jer. 5:14 — God's words feel like fire in your mouth.

Jer. 20:9 — God's words feel like burning fire in your heart.

Dan. 10:10,11 — It can make you tremble.

2 Sam. 23:2 — God's word can be sensed on your tongue.

Psalm 45:1 — Your heart can overflow with a good theme.

Ezek. 3:14 — You can feel lifted up by the Spirit and taken to another place.

1 Sam. 10:10 — It can make you prophesy.

Luke 24:32 — You can sense it as your heart burning within you.

Acts 18:5 — You can feel it as a constraining deep within.

The "Spiritual Electricity" of the Anointing Can Be Stored

The Hebrew word for "anointing" is *mischah* which means "smearing." The oil flows down from the head to the garments (Psalm 133). The Greek work for "anointing" is *charisma* which means "a rubbing in". There is a tangible impartation of the substance of the anointing upon a person when he is anointed.

Elisha's bones had so much anointing rubbed into them that when a dead man touched Elisha's dead bones, the dead man was resurrected (2 Kings 13:21)! Handkerchiefs or aprons were carried away from Paul's body to the sick, and the diseases left them and the evil spirits went out (Acts 19:12). Those who touched Jesus' garments received miracles (Mark 5:27-30; 6:56).

Inner Senses Which Detect the Holy Spirit's Movements

God has given us several senses, including the ability to "see" and "hear" and "feel", which can detect the spirit realm.

> "Truly, truly, I say to you, the Son can do nothing of Himself, unless it is something He **sees** the Father doing...I can do nothing on my own initiative. As I **hear**, I judge..." (John 5:19,30).

When we go aside to a quiet place to cultivate inner sensitivity, these are the abilities we are presenting to God and asking Him to fill. It may take quite a bit of practice to become skilled at seeing and hearing from the spirit realm. That is why God often calls us away from the normal activities of life to learn this art. Let me describe this learning process a bit as I and others have experienced it.

How to increase one's spiritual sensitivity to the Holy Spirit

"I was in the Spirit on the Lord's day, and I heard behind me a loud voice, like the sound of a trumpet, saying, 'Write in a book what you see...'" (Revelation 1:10,11).

"But solid food is for the mature, who **because of PRACTICE have their senses trained** to discern good and evil" (Heb. 5:14).

According to the Word of God, you can practice and train your spiritual senses! Quite amazing. I thought you either "had it" or you didn't. You were either a seer or you weren't. Moving in the Spirit and spiritual power can be developed and increased very much like a body builder can develop his or her body through practice. The more you do various exercises every day, the stronger you become. Granted, some start out stronger and will, therefore, probably end up stronger, but **everyone can improve to a great extent.**

I spent a year learning and practicing to see and hear. I discovered that God's voice and vision within sound like spontaneous thoughts or spontaneous impressions which "just appear", especially when I have opened my heart in faith and asked God to reveal Himself to me. I practiced looking and listening with the eyes and ears of my heart every morning during devotions. And I began doing what John did, and David and all the prophets — I began writing down what I was seeing and hearing in my journal. My learning process, struggles and experiments in these areas is described in detail in my books *Communion with God* and *Dialogue with God*. Also, see the appendix entitled "Four Keys to Hearing God's Voice" for further explanation.

At first, I was very tentative and unsure. Was the spirit world really there, or was it my imagination? Could the experiences of the Bible be true within me, or was it simply a dusty book to study and use to build theology? I had to take a leap of faith and begin to trust that God was the same yesterday, today and forever. I had to believe that Christianity was more than a creed. It is a dynamic, living relationship between me and the Lord Jesus Christ through fellowship with the Holy Spirit. I had always believed that in my head. I had just never taken it completely seriously and lived out the ramifications of that belief in the realms of my own personal experience by seeing and sensing the Holy Spirit's movements within and through me. Now, I was choosing to live it out and **experience** the stories recorded in the Bible. My rational mind fought in disbelief, so I had it go back to the Scriptures and re-read them, to become fully convinced that God had given me the **authority** to live this way. Then I had to **practice** sensing God's wonderful Holy Spirit within me and within the room. I had to learn to become sensitive to the **flow** of this river of the Holy Spirit through me. It was a battle which was fought for a long time.

I used to scoff at the artists of the Middle Ages who painted pictures of saints with a glow around their heads. How could they be so unrealistic and naive? But it is true — There is a glow, a radiation of energy which is emitted from each of us. Seers today can both see it and feel it. Kirlean photography can and has photographed it. You could begin looking for this glow that surrounds people. How intense and bright is it? Is it clear or do dark colors mar it? Put your hand near your skin. Can you feel it? How far from your skin does it go out? Are there layers to it? How does it taper off? There is a whole realm of the spirit to which we have been blind. Science is now developing more and more sensitive instruments which help us see things we have not seen before. Those who learn to use the eyes of their hearts will see and feel this world even without these instruments. You can be one of them. You can travel down this road in faith. Why not begin experimenting now and train your senses as the months and years go on? Why not learn to release the healing anointing and set people free?

Some sensations of the Spirit

Following are some of the descriptions people have given to the sensing of this flow. The following is from John Wimber.

> "Sometimes I sense God telling me to speak a word of command when praying for divine healing. The words — usually a very short sentence — come out before I consciously form them. Words of command come with a burst of faith. I feel the confidence and power of God rise in my heart and release it through my speech. Typically I lay hands near the afflicted area and say, 'I break the power of this condition in the name of Jesus,'....In some instances I speak directly to evil spirits, commanding them to leave....My hands usually tingle and are warm, and I feel something like electricity come out of them when I speak a word of command....I have come to associate feelings like tingling and heat with an anointing of the Holy Spirit on me for healing. Other examples of sensations associated with an anointing for healing include pain or heat in my body in an area that corresponds to where the person I am praying for hurts. When I pray for the person my pain disappears."[1]

"We have experienced visions functioning in divine healing. We now sometimes see (spiritually) where in a person's body the sickness is located. At other times we see a dark shadow outside of the body at the spot of the sickness. We sometimes are seeing insects, or larger animals like birds of prey, crocodiles, snakes, etc., being located either inside or outside of the body....After having prayed (a word of command) we sometimes see a kind of light over the person...just as the evil animal has disappeared. Several times we have seen something like a bright hand touching the sick spot."[2]

People's Response to the Holy Spirit

All sorts of spiritual and physical phenomena have been associated with revivals and have always raised questions in people's minds, as the body's reactions to the presence and power of the Spirit of God are not as rational and controlled as we often would like. They include falling over, shaking, trembling, sobbing, laughing, and screaming out, to name just a few. Some may also exhibit drunken actions (Acts 2), perspiration, deeper breathing, an increased pulse rate, a gentle trembling, fluttering of the eyelids, or a quiet sense of joy and peace. Some are thrown on the floor and shake or laugh for hours. When ministering deliverance as a part of healing, you may see bodily writhing and distortions in many forms as demons manifest and come out. These could include violent convulsing movements, hissing, coughing, vomiting, prolonged and loud wailing, and even demonic trance-like states as the demons leave.

Satan can, and does, counterfeit these sensations. Even Jonathan Edwards acknowledges that "as the influences of the true Spirit abounded, so counterfeits did also abound: the devil was abundant in mimicking, both the ordinary and extraordinary influences of the Spirit."[3] However, we do not throw out the true because of the counterfeit. If you search Scriptures, you will find many of these manifestations listed there also (Mark 1:21-26; 1 Sam. 1:2- 17; Acts 2:13,15; Dan. 8:17,18; 10:8-11; Acts 9:4; Ezek. 1:28; 3:23; Mark 9:20; Gen. 42:28; Ex. 19:16; Ezra 9:4; Psalm 2:11; 119:120; Isa. 66:5; Jer. 5:22; 23:9; Matt. 28:4; Mark 5:33; Luke 8:47; Acts 7:32; 16:29).

Healing Is Very Complex

Because we have a spirit, soul, and body, healing can and does occur on all three levels. Various approaches would be used on each level. In addition, Jesus included a fourth area, the area of demonization. Most people have problems on at least two levels, so various types of prayer must be used. Praying to heal past hurts is often coupled with deliverance prayer. Physical healing and deliverance prayer can often flow together. Sometimes prayers for general sins are needed. Curses may need to be broken, and confession, repentance, cleansing, and forgiveness for personal sins often occur.

You should be constantly attuned to the anointing and leading of the Holy Spirit as you minister. You can discern the Holy Spirit's movements through: 1) the leadings in your spirit; 2) what you see with the eyes of your spirit happening to the other person; 3) what you see with your natural eyes happening to the person; and 4) what the person tells you he is experiencing. **Practice** will bring increased skill in each of these abilities.

Being **mentored** by a person (or a team) who has developed skills in these areas will speed up your own personal maturation. This kind of mentor may be hard to find. Several specialists such as John Wimber, Francis MacNutt and Charles and Frances Hunter have developed videos and other teaching materials which can be used if personalized help is unavailable. Certain people have various specialties. I once sat under Mark Sanford's ministry and was astounded at his ability to reach deep into one's soul to minister healing for bitter-root judgments and expectancies. You may want to find different mentors and study and minister under them for periods of time as you master skills in various areas of spiritual sensitivity and healing ministry. I also encourage you to be part of a small group of Christians who meet regularly for prayer, worship, and ministry time. During these gatherings, practice together the things we are speaking about in this chapter.

The Prayer Model of John Wimber

Since healing is so complex, John Wimber teaches a five step methodology for healing prayer.[4]

Step One: The interview — Ask the person what they are seeking prayer for, and listen to them with your outer ears, while listening to the Holy Spirit with your inner ears. You ask, "Where does it hurt?" "What do you want me to pray for?"

Step Two: The diagnostic decision — Determine in your heart what the root of the problem is. Ask, "Why does this person have this condition?"

Step Three: The prayer selection — Determine what type(s) of prayer should be used. Ask "What kind of prayer is needed to help this person?"

Step Four: The prayer engagement — Begin ministering in prayer, staying sensitive to the Holy Spirit and keeping your eyes open so you can see any outer manifestations of the Holy Spirit. This step answers the question, "How effective are our prayers?"

Step Five: Post-prayer directions — Give any necessary homework to strengthen the gains which have been made in prayer. Answer the questions, "What should this person do to remain healed?" and "What should this person do if he or she was not healed?"

How to Increase the Flow of the Anointing During the Ministry Time

1. As you begin, quiet yourself down and become sensitive to the Holy Spirit within you. Various things can assist you, including music, stillness, relaxing, breathing deeply, fixing your eyes on Jesus, tuning to flow (spontaneity), and praying in tongues. Do what you need to do to feel connected to your innermost being and to the Holy Spirit who is joined to your spirit.

2. Repent of any and all sin. Receive the cleansing blood of Jesus over them. Make sure your heart and conscience are not condemning you.

3. Experience love ("Jesus, moved with compassion, healed..."). Oil flows when brethren dwell together in unity (Ps. 133). The power of God flows most freely when you have joined your heart in love to God, self, and the one you are praying for.

4. "After laying on hands, I pray aloud that the Holy Spirit come and minister to the person. My prayers are quite simple: 'Holy Spirit, I invite you to come on this person and release your healing power,' or 'Holy Spirit, come and show us how to pray,' or more succinctly, 'Holy Spirit, come.'"[5]

5. If you see a manifestation of the Holy Spirit's presence upon the body of the person for whom you are praying, encourage him to open his heart more fully to the Lord. You can ask the Holy Spirit to continue to pour His life out on the person. You can pray, "More of your power, Lord. More!" One fundamental principle is, "When you honor what the Lord is doing, He will usually do more."

Some specific techniques

1. Sometimes you may be unsure what the Holy Spirit is doing because you are not certain of any outer manifestations upon the person you are praying for. Or you may be uncertain about inner words and visions you are sensing. In this case you can ask the person, "Do you feel anything now, a warmth or tingling?" "Is God speaking to you?" Unfortunately, many people are insensitive to their bodies. But some may give you an affirming response which will help you identify and focus on where and how God is ministering to them.

2. You can look over the person's body, soul, and spirit with the eyes of your heart to see what you can see. Look at various parts to see what may be damaged or bound, or closed and not allowing for free flow. Ask God how to deal with what you see. I watched a skilled healing evangelist in New Zealand do this very effectively as he moved from person to person, praying for the working of the Holy Spirit in their lives. He discerned blocks in the person's heart, called them out, and prayed for the Holy Spirit to remove them. It was amazing to see the good results. It is not just a matter of doing the same thing with everyone. It is being continuously sensitive to the Holy Spirit and the person's spirit for whom you are praying and speaking forth what you are sensing.

3. One minister taught us to form groups of three or four people, encircling the one for whom we were praying. The goal is to have one person in the group who has been healed of the affliction against which you are praying because he will have faith. Another person in the group might currently have the same problem because he will have compassion. A third person in the group should be a close friend or family member because he will have love. All lay hands on the client in a soaking way, allowing a divine radiation treatment to last for 15 to 30 minutes. Sit quietly as you do this, seeing your hands as the hands of Jesus being laid upon the person and seeing the healing power of Jesus flowing into the person. Excellent results were realized.

4. John Wimber says that he determines it is time to quit praying when any of the following happen: the Holy Spirit indicates it is over, usually by withdrawing His power; he sees that the person for whom he is praying is not responding to his prayers; he no longer senses the Holy Spirit moving through him; the person indicates it is over;

he cannot think of anything else to pray for; or, he has prayed for everything and it seems that he has not gained any ground.[6]

How to increase the flow of the anointing in your daily life

You can raise the general level of anointing in your life by the practice of various Christian disciplines.

1. Practice matures and strengthens one's spiritual sensitivities (Heb. 5:14). Practice looking and listening and feeling and sensing the realm of the Holy Spirit daily.

2. Spend time praying over the Holy Scriptures, asking for and receiving spiritual revelation (Ps. 119:18,130; Eph. 1:17,18).

3. Practice abiding in Christ and praying without ceasing. For me, that means having an attitude of dependence upon Jesus and staying tuned to intuition and inner pictures, thoughts and feelings, honoring them and acting upon them.

4. "But you, beloved, **building yourselves up** on your most holy faith; praying in the Holy Spirit; keep yourselves in the love of God..." (Jude 20,21). I believe that praying **in** the Holy Spirit means that I am Spirit-sensitized as I pray — I am sensing Spirit flow, (through impressions, spontaneous words, spontaneous pictures and spontaneous feelings), and I am praying out of this leading. To pray **with** the Spirit (1 Cor. 14:14,15) means to pray in tongues. This, too, energizes one's spirit (1 Cor. 14:2,4).

5. Be constantly increasing in faith, hope and love (I Cor. 13:13). All gifts operate in proportion to one's level of faith and grace (Rom. 12:6). One can grow strong in faith, as well as increase in grace (Rom. 4:20; 2 Pet. 1:2).

Increasing the corporate anointing

If you will recall, we began by saying there were three anointings which can operate in the healing flow: the believer's anointing, the anointing for ministry, and the corporate anointing. As each of these is increased, the magnitude of healing increases. All three anointings are increased and decreased by essentially the same means.

My most exciting experience of corporate anointing was during a course on physical healing which I taught at a Bible school. Our group had been together for months, going from course to course, learning and growing together. There was total harmony and unity, a high level of faith, spirituality, and spiritual sensitivity. We began our meetings with praise and worship to charge our faith. We would then gather around and lay hands on the one being prayed for. We all looked for vision and listened for God's voice. We all led out in prayer, spoken word, or command, sharing what we were receiving. Almost everyone we prayed for was healed, including a baby dying in a hospital, who was touched by a handkerchief we all laid hands on and prayed over. It was a wonderful, super-charged experience. I hunger to live in that kind of a spiritually-charged atmosphere continuously. May God grant all of us small and large group settings where this is commonplace.

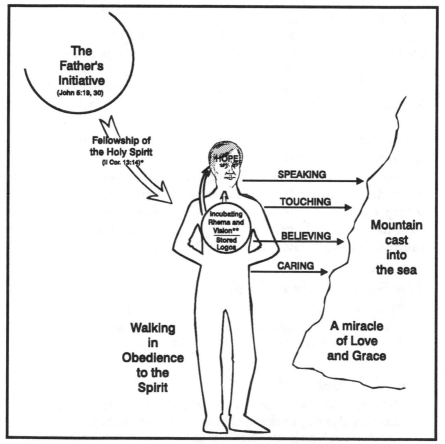

* Precipitated by: 1) being still, 2) lifting up your eyes, and 3) tuning to spontaneity.

** When the eye of your heart is clearly dwelling only on God's *rhema* and vision, your whole being is charged with His light and power (Luke 11:34-36).

Elements in the Flow of Life

The following diagram capsulizes many of the key concepts we have discussed in this chapter as they relate to releasing the flow of the healing anointing of God through us to others.

Shall We Take the Laboratory to God?

Does spiritual healing operate by laws, or is it just by chance? If there are spiritual laws behind it, can these be discovered and investigated? Could we improve our "batting average" in the area of healing prayer with more intensive experiential research into it? I think we could. I have read that there are nearly 300 such investigative studies written up. Unfortunately, the books they appear in were published through the New Age movement and not the Church, so I didn't purchase them. Perhaps it is time for leaders and/or researchers in the area of Christian healing to do some experimental research in the areas of healing prayer. Not to prove that God was right all along (which we already know), but to give us greater understanding and confidence in our experiences in the spirit realm.

If you feel a call to do this, there is a Christian book on the market which describes how to do critical research and investigative studies, setting up proper controls and control groups. You would probably want to read it and apply its principles as you set up your study. It is called *A Christian's Guide to Critical Thinking*.

The Secret of Jesus' Life

"Do you not believe that I am in the Father, and the Father in Me? The words that I speak to you I do not speak on My own authority; but the Father who dwells in Me does the works" (John 14:10).

Jesus' Prayer for Us

"That they all may be one, as You, Father, are in Me, and I in You; that they also may be one in Us, that the world may believe that You sent Me. And the glory which You gave Me I have given them, that they may be one just as We are one; I in them, and You in Me; that they may be made perfect in one, and that the world may know that You have sent Me, and have loved them as You have loved Me" (John 17:21-23).

May our lives fulfill His prayer, and may a healing revival fill the land.

Additional Resources

Power Healing by John Wimber — In my estimation, this is the best book I have read on how to move into a healing ministry. A must.

The Anointing of the Holy Spirit by Peter Tan — The best book I have read on how to grow in the anointing.

Healing by Francis MacNutt — Excellent book on healing.

The Power to Heal by Francis MacNutt — Excellent follow up book.

How to Heal the Sick by Charles and Frances Hunter — Excellent book on healing.

Handbook for Healing by Charles and Frances Hunter — Excellent!

How to Live and Not Die by Norvel Hayes — Excellent!

Healing Through Spiritual Warfare by Dr. Peggy Scarborough — Excellent!

Communion With God by Mark and Patti Virkler — Trains you how to become sensitive to the voice and vision of God.

Dialogue With God by Mark and Patti Virkler — Same as above, but shorter, and more a story format.

Naturally Supernatural by Mark and Patti Virkler — Teaches how to live sensitized to the Spirit's flow within.

Abiding in Christ by Mark and Patti Virkler — Same themes as *Naturally Supernatural*; however, in more a workbook form and more extensive.

The Flow of Life by Mark and Patti Virkler — A list of all New Testament references to "power" separated into the categories of *exousia, dunamis* and *energes*, plus more.

A Christian's Guide to Critical Thinking by Dr. Henry Virkler. Dr. Henry Virkler is my brother, and this is an excellent book teaching Christians how to set up a valid scientific research study. If you are planning to do a research project in the area of prayer and healing prayer (or any area), get this book and follow the principles therein.

References

[1] Wimber, John, *Power Healing* (New York: Harper and Row, 1987), p. 208.

[2] Wimber, p. 209.

[3] Wimber, p. 213.

[4] Wimber, pp. 199-235.

[5] Wimber, p. 212.

[6] Wimber, p. 234.

Chapter 12

The Healing Value of Fasting

God says that when you engage in a proper fast,

"...thine health shall spring forth speedily..." (Isa. 58:8).

The Bible says that fasting promotes health! Why would that be? The answer is not too hard to discover. We have already learned that your body will heal itself if you give it the opportunity to do so. Specifically, we said, you need to: 1) detoxify your body, 2) build your immune system, and 3) nourish your cells. Which of these is being done when you fast?

To start with, you are not taking in any foods which contain toxins so your body has a greatly reduced intake of foreign matter to deal with. Secondly, the process of digestion is quite a bit of work, involving many bodily functions. The activities involved in digestion are greatly reduced, or eliminated altogether on a fast in which you are only drinking water. This gives your body more energy to divert to other activities since so much energy is not being consumed in the digestion process. Increased energies can be put into your immune system as it works to detoxify your body and rebuild and refurbish various areas.

Did you notice that in the above verse, it does not say that fasting heals your body? It says your **health will spring forth**. Wow! **Our bodies do the healing** — it springs up from within our bodies. So we would not say that fasting heals. We would say that fasting prepares the way to allow your body to heal itself in a much more rapid manner than it normally can. "**Speedily**" is the word the Bible uses. Not bad! Perhaps if I am sick, one of the first things I might want to do is to give my body a break and fast for a few days and see if my health didn't speedily spring forth. Who knows? The Bible just might be right! God might just know something about doctoring after all! That is hard to believe since He has not had access to twentieth century medical testing laboratories. Do you think His approach might be too old-fashioned, or do you think His method might be an outstanding idea?

I guess I never thought about it; I just assumed that modern medicine was more effective than fasting. I would always go to a doctor when I became ill. I never tried fasting when sick to see what might happen. However, after I thought about it for a bit, read a few books on fasting for health purposes, and experimented with it on my own body, I decided to change my mind. Fasting will be a **primary resort** for healing for me. (Or, perhaps, I should more correctly say that I will fast to allow my body's recuperative powers to maximize their effectiveness and allow healing to **spring forth speedily**.)

The staff at The McEachen Sanatorium in Escondido, California supervised the fasting of 715 people from 1952 to 1958, and although many of their patients did not fast as long as they would have liked them to, the results are astounding. Either great improvement or complete recovery was shown in 294 cases, while 360 experienced moderate benefit, and 61 reported no improvement.[1] That means 88.4 percent improved or totally recovered, which is a higher statistic, I believe, than modern medicine gives us. In addition, it is free medicine, with no side effects or complications.

Dr. William L. Esser, one of the world's leading Natural Hygienic Practitioners, has a retreat in West Palm Beach, Florida. He reported on the fasting of 156 people who collectively complained of symptoms from thirty-one medically diagnosed diseases, including ulcers, tumors, tuberculosis, sinusitis, pyorrhea, Parkinson's disease, heart disease, cancer, insomnia, gallstones, epilepsy, colitis, hay fever, bronchitis, asthma, and arthritis. The shortest fast among these 156 patients lasted five days and the longest, fifty-five. Only 20 percent of his patients fasted as long as Dr. Esser recommended; however, the results are as follows:

     113 completely recovered,

      31 partially recovered,

      12 were not helped;

      92 percent improved or totally recovered![2]

Psychiatrist Dr. Allan Cott used fasting as a treatment for schizo-phrenics and reported the following results in *Applied Nutrition in*

Clinical Practice: "Dr. Cott placed twenty-eight patients on an absolute fast at The Bracie Square Hospital in New York. All patients had been diagnosed as schizophrenic for at least five years and had not responded to standard treatment. Dr. Cott reported remarkable success in 60% of the cases."[3]

Why haven't our doctors recommended fasting when we are sick, especially Christian doctors who ought to go first to the Word of God to see what God has said about the areas of sickness and health? Unfortunately, because of our sacred/secular mind split, most of us do not go first (or ever) to the Bible to see what God has to say about our area of life. My prayer is: "God, please heal us so that we may see that 'the earth is the Lord's and **all** it contains'" (Ps. 24:1).

I began to think about fasting and health. I realized that when children are sick they don't want to eat, and you have to force them. (Perhaps we shouldn't — perhaps if they honored the instincts of their bodies they would get better faster.) When animals get sick, they don't eat for a few days, and then they are often well again. Come to think of it, when I am sick, I generally don't care to eat either. Perhaps, if I **learned to listen to what my body is telling me,** and honored its messages to me, it would instruct me how to most effectively take care of myself. Doctors of Natural Hygiene teach that if you fast when you are sick, you will: 1) recover more speedily, 2) avoid a lot of physical suffering, 3) be more in tune with your body, and 4) possibly lengthen your life. Not bad!

If fasting worked for a great many illnesses, it would be the cheapest medical care by far. It would cost you nothing. As a matter of fact, it would save you money since you wouldn't be eating food for several days until your body grew hungry, signaling you were well enough to begin taking food again. When God speaks on the issues of health and medicine, does He speak authoritatively, or should His words be taken with a grain of salt? If His pronouncements are authoritative, why haven't I been obeying them? Perhaps I am blinded by the Westernization of my mind. Perhaps my mind needs a bit of healing, also.

He has healed my mind, and this is my story. It began when I picked up intestinal parasites while ministering in Malaysia. I went to my doctor who sent me to a specialist. I eventually took in three sets of three-day stool samples for lab technicians to see if they could isolate the parasite. (Gross!) They couldn't find anything. The specialist informed me that the lab technicians probably wouldn't recognize a parasite if it jumped up and bit them. Did that give me confidence in microscopes and Western medicine! The specialist also told me there were many, many tests he could put me through, but since I wasn't losing weight and was able to live with the loose stools, he suggested I just do so. So I did for a year. Then I heard of a naturopath, Dr. Prytula, just across the border from me in Canada. I went to see him, and he put me on a ten-day fast to starve the varmints out, which we successfully did. He recommended a second fast sixty days later, as a follow-up to world of natural medicine, and the role of fasting in restoring health.

Dr. Prytula has seven years of training as a medical doctor, plus several additional years in natural medicine. He has had several articles published, one in the area of therapeutic fasting, which he has been kind enough to allow us to reprint below.

Therapeutic Fasting – by Dr. Michael A. Prytula, ND

"Most people first get exposed to fasting through their television sets. As they eat their potato chips and swig their pop, the evening news shows pictures of protesters trying to get a point across by depriving themselves of food. The protesters are usually being overdramatic in showing themselves as weak, and apathetic, after only a few days of fasting. Most people's first reaction is, 'Oh no, they are going to starve to death without food.' Starving and fasting are very different, contrary to a popular misconception.

"Most people who fast do so for either therapeutic or religious purposes. Fasting is the oldest form of therapy. It is mentioned 74 times in the Bible. Christ fasted 40 days in meditation. Hippocrates, the Father of Medicine, routinely recommended prolonged fasting. Infants, as well as animals, typically fast by refusing food when they are ill. Most people remain uninformed of the beneficial effects of fasting when sick, and continue to advise their loved one to 'eat and keep up your strength'. Nothing worse could be done to lower one's vitality in acute illness than eating.

"Fasting typically means abstinence of food and drink, except water, for a specific period of time. But there are many variations in this, depending upon what the goal of the fast is. There are fruit fasts, juice fasts, and vegetable fasts. The fasting process spares the essential tissues (e.g. vital organs) while utilizing non-essential tissue (e.g. fat) for fuel.

"Starvation is a process in which the body utilizes essential tissue for fuel. During starvation the body uses protein as a fuel source as most of the fat stores have already been depleted during the fasting phase. The protein that it uses is typically the protein structure from organs and muscle. A 160-pound man could safely fast for up to two or three months before starvation sets in.

"Although therapeutic fasting is probably one of the oldest known therapies, it has been the subject of only limited study by the scientific community. Research into fasting has been reported since 1880. The medical journals have since carried articles on the use of fasting in the treatment of diabetes, mental diseases, skin conditions, obesity, arthritis, chemical poisoning, and others.

"In 1950, at the University of Minnesota, 32 volunteers fasted for up to eight months while detailed observations were made. These findings were compared to food deprivation observations which were made during the Second World War. The researchers found that fasting did not cause vitamin or mineral deficiencies, and that skin diseases and diabetes improved.

"In 1984, in a random trial of 88 patients with acute pancreatitis, fasting was determined to be the treatment of choice. The finding was that neither nasogastric suction (a surgical technique), nor cimetidine (pharmaceutical drug), offer any advantage over fasting alone in the treatment of mild to moderate acute pancreatitis of any etiology.

"*The American Journal of Industrial Medicine*, in 1984, studied patients who had ingested rice oil contaminated with PCB's. After undergoing seven- to ten-day fasts, all patients reported improvement in symptoms, and some reported dramatic relief of symptoms. This research supported past research of PCB-poisoned patients, and indicates the therapeutic effects of fasting. However, caution must be used with patients known to suffer significant contamination with fat-soluble toxins. As an example, DDT is mobilized during a fast and may reach blood levels toxic to the nervous system.

"There have been many other studies that have been done and have reported significant findings. But unfortunately fasting, as with most natural therapies, cannot be patented. Therefore, making fasting an industry is not a worthwhile investment. Hence, in spite of all its positively reported benefits, it remains a very poorly researched therapy.

"The question most people ask is what can they expect. For the first few days (anywhere from three to ten days) most people feel ill. This occurs because of their bodies' shift in metabolic processes, from assimilation of food to elimination. As our body mobilizes toxic materials, either stored in the liver or in fat cells, into the blood stream, the organs of elimination typically cannot handle the work load to which they are being subjected. Until this backlog of toxic materials is metabolized and eliminated, the person feels ill. This is commonly referred to as a healing crisis. After the healing crisis has subsided, the person fasting notices a stronger increase in energy, clear-headedness, and a stronger sense of well being. In some who meditate or pray, a euphoria can be experienced (this is commonly what the religious benefits of fasting are used for).

"The second most popular question is, "Will I feel hungry?" Most people notice that they are intensely hungry for the first few days, followed by almost no hunger at all. But for those few people who attach a much higher social and psychological stigma to food, it can be very hard.

"In reading this article, you might think only people with diseases should fast. I often recommend fasting to people who want to prevent diseases from occurring, or high-powered business executives who want to increase their productivity. Everyone should fast periodically to maintain optimum functioning and optimum health. For at least the first fast, you should consult with a licensed practitioner who is well-versed in fasting and its protocols."

Spiritual Benefits of Fasting

Dr. Prytula's article above offers an excellent overview of the physical benefits of fasting for health. Now let's turn to Isaiah 58:6-12 and see some additional **spiritual benefits** of a fast which is done with the proper attitudes.

> "Is not this the fast that I have chosen? to loose the bands of wickedness, to undo the heavy burdens, and to let the oppressed go free, and that ye break every yoke? Is it not to deal thy bread to the hungry, and that thou bring the poor that are cast out to thy house? when thou seest the naked, that thou cover him; and that thou hide not thyself from thine own flesh? Then shall thy light break forth as the morning, and thine health shall spring forth speedily: and thy righteousness shall go before thee; the glory of the LORD shall be thy reward. Then shalt thou call, and the LORD shall answer; thou shalt cry, and he shall say, Here I am. If thou take away from the midst of thee the yoke, the putting forth of the finger, and speaking vanity; And if thou draw out thy soul to the hungry, and satisfy the

afflicted soul; then shall thy light rise in obscurity, and thy darkness be as the noon day: And the LORD shall guide thee continually, and satisfy thy soul in drought, and make fat thy bones: and thou shalt be like a watered garden, and like a spring of water, whose waters fail not. And they that shall be of thee shall build the old waste places: thou shalt raise up the foundations of many generations; and thou shalt be called, The repairer of the breach, The restorer of paths to dwell in."

What an awesome list of benefits of a proper fast! I fasted often during my twenties and early thirties for spiritual purposes, but never for personal physical healing. And from age thirty-two to forty I pretty much quit fasting altogether. Coincidentally(?), by age thirty-six my health was breaking down.

Let's go back and finish my story of Dr. Michael Prytula putting me on a seven-day distilled water fast, during which I also drank a bit of natural medicine called Bentonite (available in health stores), which was designed to help scrub down my stomach and intestines. We did starve out about 95 percent of the varmints in my intestines, and my gastrological problems of two years disappeared as a result of the fast! Talk about happy! My hat went off to Dr. Prytula and natural medicine, and my exploration of natural medicines began.

However, the best part of this story is still to be told. I discovered during my first two bowel movements after the fast that I not only discharged the burned-out junk from my intestines, I, at the same time, discharged all the spiritual oppression with which I had been struggling. I was healed spiritually and emotionally, as well as physically!

I had been struggling with a lot of oppression for about three years. I felt worse than at any time in my twenty-five years as a Christian. I felt hostile, dominant, alienated, fearful, discouraged, suicidal, you name it. If it is a negative emotion, I had been fighting it continuously for three years. I would bind satan and rebuke him in Jesus' name and feel pressure lift somewhat for about five minutes, and then it would settle back down again. To give you a brief glimpse of the agony of my soul during those years, I excerpt the following characteristic section from my journal.

"I have been feeling anger, rejection, and bitterness grow within me over the last two years. My spirit has become sour; I am full of hostility. My body is heavy spiritually, physically, and emotionally. I am down and depressed. My back is out of place, and will not go in and stay in, my neck has hurt for three months, my toe is inflamed. I am a wreck in every way. I have wanted to leave everything for the last two years."

That is as bad as some of David's psalms. It makes it crystal-clear that nothing good dwells in me other than the Holy Spirit, and that without His anointing and His healing, I have no life.

Several emotional traumas had occurred just before this period of my life which contributed to the mess I was in. You know, being healed once is no guarantee that more hurts will not come down the pike and force you back to the everlasting arms of Jesus for healing again and again.

Let me share my journaling that occurred about two days after the fast was over.

"I have been healed by God working through the seven-day fast."

"Yes, Mark, that is entirely right. You have been healed by Me, working through this seven-day fast. You have been healed emotionally, spiritually, and physically. Now walk in My health that nothing worse befall you."

"Thank You, Lord. Help strengthen me, I pray."

"Strengthen Thyself through the reading of My Word and through prayer in My Spirit and you shall be whole."

"Yes, Lord."

"Read Isaiah 58 now." (I read it and concluded that the Lord has performed Isaiah 58 for me this day as a result of seeking Him through this seven-day fast.)

"Yes, Mark, I have. I have broken the bands of wickedness which have bound you. I have set the captive free. I have broken every bond.

"Your light will break out like the dawn, and your recovery will speedily spring forth, and your righteousness will go before you, the glory of the Lord will be your rear guard, you will call and I will answer. You will cry, and I will say, 'Here I am.'

"Now be careful to remove legalism, criticism, backbiting, and, generally speaking, wickedness. Give yourself to those who are hungry spiritually, and satisfy those who have been afflicted through religion, and your light will rise in the darkness, and your gloom will be totally healed, and I will continually guide you and satisfy your desire in scorched places, and give strength to your bones (i.e. give you long health), and you will be refreshed and you will be a continuing fountain of water, and you will rebuild the ancient ruins within Christianity. You will restore truths lost for generations of time. You will establish new spiritual foundations upon which they may build, and you will be called the repairer of the breach — the one who built a bridge back to the original foundations, and the restorer of paths, or tracks, upon which people could walk spiritually.

"You will be Mine, saith the Lord of Hosts, because I have chosen you before the foundations of the earth to prepare the way of the Lord. Even as John was a voice crying in the wilderness, so you, too, shall be a voice crying from the wilderness, prepare ye the way of the Lord. And many shall come out to the wilderness to see you and to hear you. And what is it they have gone out to see? A man clothed in rich honor? A man clothed with titles and degrees? No, they have come out to see one filled with the power of the Spirit, an anointed teacher of My Word. That is what they have come out to see. One clothed in the power of the Spirit. That is what they have come out to see.

"Mark, receive your commission and walk ye in it, saith the Lord of Hosts."

"Lord, I receive. Anoint me and I shall give You all praise and glory for that which You do through me."

Why Do I Share All This?

I share all this with you for several reasons. I know from talking to people across the nation, especially pastors, that I am not the only one struggling with spiritual and physical oppression. I trust my story will touch others and give them insight into how to be healed.

I am astounded at how radically this seven-day distilled water fast healed me, emotionally and spiritually. It is the difference between night and day. It is like being saved again. I believe the Bible teaches that we may all experience such healing through proper Biblical fasting.

Reflections on other fasts I have taken

This success with fasting caused me to reflect back on other fasts which I have been on during my life. One was a 40-day liquid fast (i.e. we included juices, milk, and water) which Patti and I went on in our early twenties. We were seeking spiritual breakthrough in the release of healing power, having just become charismatic. At the close of this fast, I prayed for a cancer patient in Roswell Hospital in Buffalo who had many tumors and many other ailments. His healing began the day I prayed for him. His bed sores, which had not been healing, began healing that day. He had not been able to keep food down. That day he did for the first time. And although he was expected to die within days, his health returned, and he was released from the hospital and once again walked the streets of his city. It was a rather dramatic healing, as the doctors expected him to die within days. It left me convinced that indeed God's power could flow through me, so I pressed on into becoming a full-fledged charismatic. Another benefit of that fast was to lose twenty-five pounds, the only other time until recently that I have been down to weight in my adult life. Awesome!

Other fasts of various lengths including one-day, three-day, seven-day, and ten-day, have brought great release in my life spiritually. Following is a note from my journal after listing twenty things God had shown me during a ten-day fast:

> "Maybe most important, I have seen that the way to **real life changes** is through taking several days alone with God in prayer and fasting, allowing Him to speak into my life, obeying His words, clinging to His strength, and receiving **rebirth** within the areas He is changing. This process seems to bring personal spiritual growth in a way seldom achieved through other means.

> "I need to instruct the congregation in the value of this and provide ways and places for them to experience it."

I noted that John Wesley required his pastors to fast two days a week until 3:00 in the afternoon, so what I have done generally for the last twenty years is fast breakfast and eat about 12:30 every day. I have just orange juice and vitamins in the morning and have a clearer, more alert mind, I believe, in the morning because my stomach is not digesting food. I did ask Dr. Prytula if this was all right, and his response was that orange juice makes one's system acidic, and therefore puts stress on it, and that it would be better to take apple juice and vitamins. And it would be best in the winter months to add some oatmeal also.

How Helpful Would Fasts Be in Twelve-Step Programs?

I believe in twelve-step programs, inner healing and deliverance, yet I have noticed we have not generally been proponents of extended water-fasts in many of these ministries. Should we be? Would we see dramatic things happen in these people's lives regularly, if water-fasts were a part of the programs? Will a seven-day water-fast accomplish as much as a year of counseling? I don't know. It did for me. (Perhaps a less drastic form using some fruit juices would be as effective.)

I would like to suggest this: If you are struggling with bonds that need to be broken, and you have done the normal things like praying and rebuking and confessing and memorizing and a one- or two-day liquid fast, and these have not worked, then you might want to get out the heavy artillery. I suggest that an extended water-fast (three to seven days) may be helpful.

During the Fast

During the fast, we seek God in prayer for healing, release, and deliverance. I usually feel low energy, weary, and somewhat down emotionally during the fast (unless the fast is more than seven to ten days). It is after the fast that the release is generally manifested. It is like a death and resurrection experience for me. Read Isaiah 58 in preparation, and try to keep your work load lighter during the fast, if possible. This is sometimes difficult. If you are fasting for physical health reasons, there are fasting clinics you can go to where you will be supervised. For more information, contact Victoria Bidwell, The Christian Natural Hygiene Association of America, c/o GetWell, StayWell, America, 4390 Bidwell Drive, Fremont, CA 94538. Or you can contact American Natural Hygiene Society, P.O. Box 30630, Tampa, FL 33630. 813-855-6607.

I asked Dr. Michael Prytula, ND., about the best length of a fast. He recommends three- and seven-day fasts. Much more cleansing occurs in a seven-day fast. Actually, if one is taking Bentonite (available from health food stores) during the fast, a seven-day fast has the same physical cleansing value as a seventeen-day water-fast. The following is a brief overview of how his recommended three- or seven-day colon cleanse program works: Drink four or five glasses per day of distilled water. In addition, drink four or five bentonite cleansing drinks. (Place one-half to one inch of pineapple, grape, orange, or other unsweetened fruit juice in the bottom of your glass, add 8 oz. of distilled water, and one tablespoon of hydrated bentonite. Shake well and drink immediately.)

To keep your metabolism from getting messed up, you need to use the following procedure when coming off the fast:

Day 1 — Eat only fruits and clear soups, and take acidophilus.

Day 2 — Eat same as day 1 and include vegetables.

Day 3 — Eat same as day 2 and include grains.

Day 4 — Eat same as day 3 and include fish and chicken.

Day 5 — Regular diet (trying to stay away from dairy products).

Note: If you are doing a three-day rather than a seven-day fast, you can shorten the time it takes to come off the fast to two- and-a-half days by condensing the schedule to half days, rather than one day, increments.

NOTE: PREGNANT/OR BREAST-FEEDING WOMEN AND INDIVIDUALS WITH SUGAR METABOLISM PROBLEMS SHOULD NOT FAST.

Do not be surprised if you feel poorly during the first few days of a fast. Your body will be eliminating toxic wastes that may have been stored since your birth. During the cleanse, take things slow and easy, do not work out, and do try to relax.

A Pre-Packaged Fourteen-Day Colon Cleanse

There is a fourteen-day colon-cleanse program, developed by Dr. Albert Zehr, which involves four days of fasting in the middle of it. For the first seven days of the program, you take about nine capsules which loosen any encrusted build-up of matter on the inside of your intestines and prepare it to come off during and after the fast. After the seven days of colon preparation, you fast four days while taking some additional cleansing capsules and a form of bentonite. (Bentonite is actually clay in liquid form. You know the drawing capacities of clay. That is why it has traditionally been put on bee stings.) The final three days involve taking acidophilus, cascara, sagrada, alfalfa, and digestive enzymes. Dr. Albert Zehr packages this entire fourteen-day colon cleanse with complete instructions for easy use. Many people I know (including myself) have tried it with excellent cleansing results and health benefits. I believe it gives me various health benefits commonly associated with longer fasts, even though the fast lasts only four days. You may choose to try it.

Some Questions and Answers

Q. What kinds of fasts are there?

A. There are three basic categories of fasts. One category is the total fast in which one abstains from all food and all drink. The longest such fast in the Bible is three days. Your body cannot go without water for longer than three days.

Another category of fasts is the partial fast, such as Daniel took where he abstained from bread, meat, and wine for twenty-one days (Dan. 10:3). In a partial fast, a person decides to limit the kinds of food he takes in.

The final category of fasts is called the "absolute fast", commonly called the "water-fast", wherein one abstains from all food and drinks only water. It is technically not correct to call this a water-fast because to fast means "to abstain". In a true "water-fast" one would actually be abstaining from water, which is not what is really meant. The longest absolute fast in the Bible is forty days (Luke 4).

Q. Is all fasting to be private?

A. Not necessarily. There are many proclaimed fasts for corporate spiritual purposes found in the Bible (Ezra 8:21- 23,31,32; 1 Sam. 31:11,13; 2 Chron. 20:3; 1 Sam. 14:24; Acts 13:1-3).

Q. How do I know when to quit fasting?

A. You will get hungry again. After about three days of fasting, your hunger pains subside and will not return until your body has burned off all excess fat and detoxified. When it comes to the point of beginning to burn off tissue from vital organs, it will signal you with severe hunger pains. You should quit fasting immediately.

Q. What else might happen on a fast?

A. As part of your detoxifying, you may have foul breath and foul body orders. Your tongue is likely to become coated. Weakness may occur during the first several days. Then energy and health is likely to replace it. Sickness and tumors can, and do, disappear during fasting.

Q. How much weight will I lose?

A. Most people lose about a pound per day, a bit more during the first few days, and less than that as time goes on. Fasting is not the best way to lose weight. The better way is to eat the Genesis diet and exercise.

Q. Should thin people fast?

A. One reason some people are too thin is that their bodies are not properly assimilating the food they eat. A fast can cleanse and detoxify their bodies, so they begin functioning properly after the fast, and they begin putting on weight. Obviously, during the fast they will lose weight.[4]

Q. Can fasting help me live to over 100?

A. There are 32,000 centenarians currently alive in the United States. The Bible says that "The life of the flesh is in the blood" (Lev. 17:11). Fasting helps keep the blood clean and thus enhances life. Dr. Alexis Carrel of the Rockefeller Institute kept a chicken heart alive for twenty-eight years by simply changing the fluid in which it lived every day. As long as toxins were removed and nutrients provided, the cells continued to live. Only when an attendant forgot to change the fluid one day, did the chicken heart die. Dr. Carrel declared:

> "The cell is immortal. It is merely the fluid in which it floats that degenerates. Renew this fluid at proper intervals, and give the cell nourishment upon which to feed, and so far as we now, the pulsation of life may go on forever."[5]

Q. Should I fast periodically?

A. Yes. Jesus expected that we would. He said, "WHEN you fast..." (Matt. 6:16-18). He didn't say, "IF you fast." So you should discern an approach to fasting which keeps you in tip top shape physically and spiritually. Derek Prince, an anointed teacher who has been very influential in my life, fasted one day per week. I have tried many schedules of fasting throughout my life. I suggest you experiment and discover what is best for you. It may change as you go along. Be open and flexible. Listen to your body and listen to your spirit. When either of them says, "I need a fast", honor that. It may be better to do that than to have a precise schedule. I prefer grace to law. The danger is, of course, that you allow your grace to become license, and say, "Now that I don't have a schedule for fasting, I guess my body really never wants a fast, so I will just skip fasting altogether." If you can operate with integrity under grace, it may be the preferred way to go.

Q. Why don't many churches teach about fasting?

A. Because of ignorance. One seminary student published the results of the research required for his graduate degree. He sent a questionnaire to over three hundred church leaders. One question was "Do you think that fasting would develop your Christian life?"

55 replied, "Yes."

32 replied "No."

83 were uncertain.[6]

Q. Can children fast?

A. Sure. They will desire to naturally when they are sick. As long as they are listening to their bodies, and under adult supervision, they can fast without it hurting them.

Q. Who should not fast?

A. Anyone fearful of fasting, people who are extremely emaciated, weak, or in extreme degeneration. People who have inactive kidneys or any type of kidney disease, or a bad or damaged liver. (Too many toxins can enter the bloodstream at once and the liver and kidneys are not able to handle it). Pregnant and breast-feeding women, and people taking insulin should not fast.

Q. What about rest during a fast?

A. Try, as much as possible, to get increased physical, mental, and emotional rest.

Additional Resources

Fast Your Way To Health by Lee Bueno. This book has my highest recommendation. It is very current, well-written, instructional, informative, and has a balance between the physical and spiritual benefits of fasting.

Fasting Can Save Your Life by Herbert M. Shelton. Herbert Shelton has supervised over 40,000 fasts for health purposes. Eighteen chapters of his book deal with healing eighteen different diseases through fasting, plus there are an additional eighteen chapters providing general instruction on fasting. Over 450,000 copies sold.

God's Chosen Fast by Arthur Wallis. A classic on the spiritual aspects of fasting. Highly recommended.

Healthy Steps by Albert Zehr. Chapter Four details the fourteen-day colon cleanse involving the four-day fast. Chapter 14 discusses the ability of clay to heal. (Bentonite is a form of liquid clay which is taken internally as part of his fourteen-day cleanse.)

Fasting Response Form

Mark & Patti,

I would like to help you compile your study on the benefits of fasting. You may utilize the following results in your research.

Name _____ Phone _____

Address _____

City_____ State _____ Zip _____

Reason for the fast _____

_____

_____

_____

Type of fast ___ Water ___ Liquid ____ Partial diet

Length of fast _____

Results of fast _____

_____

_____

_____

_____

_____

_____

Comments: _____

_____

_____

_____

_____

_____

_____

_____

References

[1] Bueno, Lee, *Fast Your Way to Health* (Springdale, PA: Whitaker House, 1991), p. 94.

[2] Bueno, p. 95.

[3] Bricklin, Mark, *The Practical Encyclopedia of Natural Healing* (Emmaus, PA: Rodale Press, 1976), pp. 174, 175, as cited by Bueno, p. 95.

[4] Shelton, Herbert, *Fasting Can Save Your Life* (Tampa, FL: American Natural Hygiene Society, Inc., 1978, 1991), p. 77ff.

[5] Tanner, Henry, *The Fasting Story II* (Mokelumne Hill, CA: Health Research), p. 47, which is a quote by Dr. Alexis Carrel, famous biologist of the Rockefeller Institute, as cited by Bueno, p. 111.

[6] Bueno, p. 184.

Chapter 13

Tissue Cleansing

"A healing crisis is an acute reaction resulting from the ascendancy of Nature's healing forces over disease conditions. Its tendency is toward recovery, and it is, therefore, in conformity with nature's constructive principle." (from a catechism of Naturopathy)[1]

"A healing crisis is the result of an industrious effort by every organ in the body to eliminate waste products and set the stage for regeneration."[2]

Another descriptive, less threatening, phrase for "healing crisis" is "tissue cleansing."

Essentially, this is an overall picture of what happens. As we live life, we may treat our bodies in damaging ways with poor nutrition, junk food, excessive chemicals and pollutants, devitalized foods, etc. Our bodies deteriorate and sickness overcomes them. We then seek to ward off the symptoms of the sickness, not by building up our bodies' defense system (i.e. lymph system, cellular vitality, elimination system), but instead with the use of synthetic, pharmaceutical drugs which may repress the symptoms but, often, also weaken the entire body and leave the sickness undercover in our bodies. At the same time, the antibiotic drugs destroy healthy bacteria in the intestines, causing the intestinal flora to change from acidophilus to bacillus coli, further weakening the body by moving us toward autointoxication.

Now we may think we are healthy, but we are actually walking around with a weakened, sickly body which has suppressed symptoms within it. Those Americans who are still living unconsciously in the areas of diet and health are living with suppressed sicknesses and toxins within their bodies. These cause all sorts of degenerative symptoms and pains. For example, some people find that as they grow older their bodies become more sensitive to allergies, asthma, arthritis, and many other sensitivities and sicknesses. There is a reason for this: Their bodies' immune systems are breaking down, or are simply overloaded with too many toxins and damaged cells to effectively remove them all. There are too many repressed things below the surface which the immune system is trying to cope with.

As you begin to live in a healthy manner, appropriating many of the concepts within this book, you will discover over a year's time that you will regain a new healthy body. (Most cells in your body are replaced within one year). As your body gains strength and the blood becomes purer and the cells stronger and the organs cleansed, your body comes to the point where it is ready to throw off (or out) the repressed disease (or toxins) left over within your system. As your body makes this industrious move, a tissue cleansing occurs. Tissue cleansing may last from one to three days or even longer. During the tissue cleansing, you may feel the symptoms of the sickness once again as it is being discharged from your body.

Understanding Autointoxication

Autointoxication is defined as "The poisoning of the body, or some part of the body, by toxic matter generated therein."[3] The Western diet consisting of excessive protein, fats, and cholesterol and insufficient fiber causes food to remain in the intestines for many days, rather than passing through quickly (within eighteen hours) as it was supposed to do. When this happens, the foods putrefy and are then absorbed through the intestinal walls, back into our bodies, poisoning our entire system. This absolutely must stop if one is to regain vibrant health. The diet must be changed from meat and dairy products to starches, fruits, and vegetables. Enzymes must be present with the foods we eat, the intestines cleared through some elimination process, and acidophilus flora restored to the intestines. **This becomes the foundation upon which health can be built.**

Understanding the Steps into Chronic Disease

Chronic disease doesn't just happen. It is developed over years of abuse to one's body and suppression of our bodies' natural elimination responses. For example, let's start with the common cold. During a cold, the body is eliminating catarrh, phlegm, and mucus. If we mask these symptoms through the use of a drug or suppressant, we drive these substances back into our bodies and they settle in some weak organ. We are now on our way to a chronic disease.

The next suppression-symptom is the flu. If we treat it with antibiotics and penicillin, we continue to cause suppression. In addition, the use of these antibiotics destroys the friendly acidophilus flora in our intestines, once again lowering our bodies' ability to get rid of toxic materials.

The next thing that develops is hay fever. We are going up the ladder, **making** a chronic disease. Now we take antihistamines to suppress the hay fever. Next comes asthma.

Understanding the Steps Toward Healing

If the person above is going to be healed of asthma, he will have to retrace his steps using Hering's Law of Cure: "All disease is cured from within out; from the head down; and in reverse order as the symptoms have appeared." In order to rid the body of the tissue built from injurious living habits — tissue that holds disease symptoms lying latent in chronic tissue — the retracing process, the tissue cleansing, is necessary.

A child on a good health routine may experience a tissue cleansing in seven to fourteen days. For adults, the tissue cleansing usually happens after three months on a good health routine. It generally lasts about three days, starting with slight pain and discomfort which may become more severe until the point of complete expulsion has been reached. If the energy of the patient is low, the crisis sometimes lasts for a week or more.

The tissue cleansing will likely come without warning. Usually you are feeling better than you have felt in a long time. Your body is now strong enough to expel the rest of the toxic tissue, replacing it with new vitalized tissue. The old has spent itself and the new, built from life-giving foods and health-building processes, has grown stronger than the old, abused tissue. Tissue that has been built from devitalized, chemicalized food will someday have to fight with new tissue created from natural, healthy food. It is plain to see which will dominate. This is why the tissue cleansing is actually a blessing in disguise.

During the tissue cleansing, you may re-experience the disease symptoms, but there is a **very important distinction**: You continue to have natural bowel movements. The difference between a tissue cleansing and when you actually have a sickness is that when sick, bowel movements often become irregular. (Actually enemas ought to be taken if sick and your bowel movements are irregular. This will aid in elimination of toxic wastes.) Though it may feel like a disease crisis, it will not last as long or develop into another disease.

During tissue cleansing there may be an absence of appetite. Follow your body's natural cravings. Drink some extra water to aid in the detoxification. Rest both mentally and physically. Continue whatever things strengthen your body and aid in elimination. Work with your body during this crisis.

If at all possible, do not chemically suppress the symptoms which appear during a tissue cleansing. Resorting to antihistamines or other artificial suppressants only drives the poisons back into the tissues of your body, eventually causing a negative reaction elsewhere. Dr. Jensen states, "I have said so many times — if you suppress or don't allow a discharge to continue until you are clean inside, you will develop a growth."[4]

Tissue cleansing is not accomplished by either a doctor or the patient. The body's processes accomplish it. The intelligence within the body knows when tissue structure repair and regeneration is at the proper point to aggressively remove unwanted damaged tissues, and the tissue cleansing occurs.

Let's listen to Dr. Bernard Jensen, D.C. Nutritionist, describe the tissue cleansing:

> "A crisis comes usually after you feel your best. It is the will of nature. No doctor, no patient, no food, can bring a crisis on. It comes when your body is ready. It does it in its own time. It goes through slow or fast according to the patient's constitution, nervous system and what you have earned so that it will come on. You **earn** this crisis through hard work. It comes through a sacrifice, giving up bad habits, taking a new path, cleaning up the act that you've been in when your life wasn't working with the laws of nature. A crisis can come harsh, small, violently, softly, according to what is possible for the body to control and take care of. Some crises come in backaches, skin rashes, teeth can become on edge, a diarrhea can develop, joint pains can come. I have seen people have all of these symptoms, however, they do not usually come at the same moment but move from one part of the body to another or wherever the body is placing its energy for cleansing, rejuvenation and getting rid of the old tissue and acids that probably have accumulated over a period of years."[5]

It is likely that some mental conditions in people are nothing more than a toxic condition that settled in the brain areas and interferes with the proper brain and nerve activity. If your eyes are bad, maybe they are toxic. If you cannot hear, perhaps you have too much toxic material in your body. It is possible that every cell and every organ in your body needs rejuvenation. All blood cells are new every thirty days. Clean blood can then go to work cleansing every organ in your body. If you change the way you live and choose a path of health, within a year many conditions within your body will very likely clear up.

An Example of Tissue Cleansing in Action

In the book *Fast Your Way to Health*, Lee Bueno tells of her own remarkable tissue cleansing which saved her life. You should get her book if for nothing more than just this one story. It is told in the first two chapters of her book. In brief, her story goes like this: Within days of having some dental work done, she began suffering severe pain throughout her head. After several days of increasing intensity, she was forced to visit a doctor who told her she had "rheumatoid vasculitis" which is sometimes called "temporal arthritis." It affects the entire circulatory system in the body and especially impairs the main artery leading up to the brain. Allergies cause these rheumatoid diseases. She was told that it was incurable and she must learn to cope with it. The doctor encouraged her to avoid driving, flying, and singing, and offered her cortisone, which she refused.

She went to other doctors for a second, third, and fourth opinion, and they all confirmed the diagnosis. She would go blind or die if she didn't take their drugs, which, they admitted, were only a temporary solution. She asked all four doctors if her trip to the dentist could have anything to do with her problem. They all told her no. Yet a voice in her head kept saying, "Yes".

She decided to go on a professionally supervised fast at a retreat center to see if fasting would heal this incurable disease. As her fast progressed, the pain in her head intensified, until constant pain and discomfort prevailed. The director explained to her that fasting people should not suppress pain with aspirin or prescription drugs, but rather let the body heal itself. Pain is a friend, showing that healing is taking place.

After three weeks, she broke her fast and awoke the next morning with bloodshot eyes and pain that had dropped from the side to the back of her head. She was panic stricken and called her husband who prayed with her over the phone and comforted her. The director at the retreat house asked her if the pain she felt then was similar to the pain she felt when the problem first developed. In thinking back over the weeks, Lee recalled that this was exactly the location that the pain first appeared in her head. Her tissue cleansing was almost over.

Over the next two days, she ate six small, healthy meals of raw fruits and vegetables, and continued to rest. This helped her body continue its detoxifying process until, by the end of the next day, her eyes had cleared and the pressure pain had disappeared from her head. All that was left was a slight twitching sensation on the left side of her face. That, too, was a detoxifying symptom. Driving home from the retreat center, she tuned her radio to a local talk show and heard a dentist explain to a frightened caller an answer that also gave Lee understanding of what had happened to her.

The dentist explained that if a dental patient has a history of rheumatic fever (which Lee did have), the attending dentist should give an antibiotic to prevent infection before he begins. An infected tooth directs the infection into the head or even into other areas of the body. This infection most often goes straight to the heart and can result in sudden death. Or, the infection can lodge in the brain cavity and cause inflammation there.

The revelation was complete. The tissue cleansing was understood, right down to the twitching and numbness of the check which was part of the leftover Novocain being expelled from her body.

My Personal Example of a Tissue Cleansing

I experienced a tissue cleansing after one week on blue-green algae. I had prepared my intestines as instructed with several days of acidophilus capsules as well as taking enzymes with meals. With this foundation, I then began taking the Algae.

My first two days on algae nearly put me to sleep each afternoon. I suppose my body was compensating from the constant "on the go" pressure I tend to give it. The skin on my feet cracked and broke. I expect toxins were being ejected through the cracks. Then poison ivy broke out all over my body and lasted two weeks, even though I am absolutely certain I had not been near the stuff. I have always been extremely allergic to poison ivy and have had it from the top of my head to the bottom of my feet. I suspect I was experiencing suppressed toxic tissue which was finally coming out. As the poison ivy rash disappeared, aching began to fill my joints. It took me a day or two to realize that the ache was the next step in my tissue cleansing. The ache was released when I exercised. Because the exercise was empowering my lymph system, it was cleansing the joints of damaged tissues. Had I not understood the cleansing power of a tissue cleansing, and how by equipping my body with the right building blocks, it was allowed to precipitate such a cleanse, I would never have stayed on the algae. I would have felt my body was reacting negatively to the product and quit within days. However, by having insight, I pressed on. I began to feel rested after six or seven hours of sleep. In addition, I felt outstanding energy throughout the day without being on any other herbs that would stimulate my body! I was impressed that my body was getting something in blue-green algae that it really needed.

Dr. Bernard Jensen said, "The liver is probably one of the first organs we should take care of. This is the organ that detoxifies and eliminates wastes more than any other organ in the body outside of the bowel. Some foods which can help the liver [include]...chlorophyll which is one of the greatest cleansers we have."[6] I realized that blue-green algae is high in chlorophyll.

Most people who follow the blue-green algae program, building a foundation in their intestines for a week with the use of acidophilus and enzymes and then adding the algae, will experience a "tissue cleansing." I find it exciting to think of all the people who could experience improved health and vitality. I recommend it highly!

Kim Bright Cassano, a nationally recognized nutritionalist who has worked with thousands of people who take blue-green algae offered a few pieces of advice to me which I felt would be valuable to pass along. 1) The algae does not replace one's need for vitamins. 2) If you are making the transition to algae, take it easy, especially if you have some major health problems. Taking too much too fast can cause too acute a tissue cleansing, while going at a slower rate can make it more bearable. 3) If the tissue cleansing becomes too intense, cut back to half the amounts of algae consumed daily and then slowly return to a larger amount. 4) Your reactions are not contagious during a tissue cleansing. 5) Make sure to be drinking six to eight glasses of non-chlorinated water each day to aid in the detoxification process.

Tissue cleansings can occur one after another. For example, your first tissue cleansing may occur within days of being on a superfood as **surface** tissue becomes cleansed. Additional crises can occur months or even years later, as **deeper** organs within your body are cleansed.

Getting Some Counsel

I think it is important to get counsel as one goes through a tissue cleansing. When I experienced a tissue cleansing, I was nervous. I had probably a hundred poison ivy spots break out on my legs, stomach, back, and arms within two or three days. I know how rapidly this can spread on me and how severe the problem can become, so I wanted some answers and I wanted them now. Do I go to the doctor and get some prescription that will suppress the problem? Or, if this is a tissue cleansing, I don't really want to repress these symptoms. I want these latent toxins out. What do I do? I didn't know, so I did what I suggest each one of you do when you think you might be in a tissue cleansing: I got some counsel. I started by calling the person who had told me about the algae and asked if he could explain what was happening and what I should do. He had only been using the product for a month so he was not sure, so together we placed a conference call to Kim, the person who had told him about the product. She had been taking it for ten years and had many hundreds of examples to draw from. She provided me with much wise counsel which gave me the confidence I needed to press forward. In the **multitude of counselors there is safety**.

Find a person **with experience in what you are doing** who can counsel you. Tissue cleansing is, in my opinion, too scary and dangerous to face alone. SO GET YOURSELF UNDER SOME WISE EXPERI-ENCED COUNSEL SO YOU DO NOT DO ANYTHING FOOLISH OR DAMAGING!!! DID YOU HEAR THIS? I hope so, for your well being. I do not want to be responsible for anyone reading this chapter and damaging himself. If you follow the path of wise, experienced counsel from others who are IN THE KNOW you should be safe. "In the know" for me means, they have a good level of nutritional and healing knowledge and experience (preferably with an accompanying medical degree or nurses degree). Let's be wise in these matters.

Some Summary Reflections

Dr. Henry Lindlahr said, "Give me a tissue cleansing and I will cure any disease."

Hippocrates, the Father of Medicine, said, "Give me a fever and I will cure any disease."

I suspect that healing crises occur in marriages and in our ever closer walk with our Lord Jesus Christ. I suspect once we learn to look for them, we will see them rather often. Most likely, we have mistaken them for marital weakening rather than marital healing, or for increased licentiousness rather than God burning off one more level of dross in our lives. Perhaps I should "in everything give thanks." Maybe some of the "crises" in my marriage and spiritual walk are actually "healing crises".

Tissue Cleansing Worksheet

If you are doing health-oriented activities which may be precipitating a tissue cleansing, record your answer to the following question every three days.

Question: "How am I feeling?"

Day   Date of first entry below:_____
1.

3.

6.

9.

12.

15.

18.

21.

24.

27.

30.

References

[1] Jensen, Bernard. *Doctor-Patient Handbook* (Escondido, CA: Barnard Jensen Enterprises, 1976), p. 49.

[2] Jensen, *Doctor-Patient Handbook*, p. 49.

[3] Jensen, Doctor-Patient Handbook, p. 9.

[4] Jensen, Bernard. *Tissue Cleansing Through Bowel Management* (Escondido, CA: Bernard Jensen Enterprises, 1981), p. 133.

[5] Jensen, *Doctor-Patient Handbook*, p. 62.

[6] Jensen, *Doctor-Patient Handbook*, p. 45.

Chapter 14

How Do I Then Live?

Always a Learner

After reading more than seventy books on diet and health care and experimenting on my own body for ten months, I have taken the first step toward personal responsibility for my health. I still have much to learn. And I strongly suspect I shall readjust somewhat even the things that are written here as I travel along.

Some may want to argue with me. Some may want to instruct me. Some may want me to counsel them. I choose not to argue with anyone. This is not written to convince the skeptic, but to inform the searcher. I do not have time nor desire to fight with the skeptic. The one who shall teach me will be the one who is demonstrating more fruit than I have discovered. It will be the one who is living with more strength, vitality, radiance, and overall health than I am. To those I will eagerly listen. All others may hold their peace. For those who may want my counsel I prefer not to be called for personal advice, because I am not a doctor of medicine, so I cannot legally give it. If you want more insight, read the recommended books at the end of the chapters, and apply their teachings and insights as you seek the face of God and counsel of natural health specialists for final confirmation. I would avoid the counsel of doctors not trained in nutrition and preventive medicine. Their recommendation will probably involve radical invasion of your body through surgery, radiation, and caustic drugs. You most likely will want to choose more natural means.

Today we can decide how much we want to know and understand. We can live with second grade understanding or twelfth grade or even beyond. It is truly a new day. Growth usually comes slowly and with difficulty. For some it will be quick because a crisis forces immediate action. If each of us would choose to pursue the path of life, wholeness, and truth with a passion, life itself would be a more enjoyable experience. I chose to meander along for 20 years in ignorance about the proper care of my body. Now I am choosing conscious understanding and honest living. The result for me has been renewed life, vigor, vitality, energy, clarity, passion, health, and zest. These rewards have been motivation enough to urge me on. I trust I will never turn back to my old ways. I pray that you, too, choose to take responsibility for your own health. No one cares about it as much as you do. For yourself, for your family, please — choose LIFE!

We All Need Motivation to Make the Change

There are a good many things which could be motivating factors in your decision to embark on a new (actually old), more natural way of living.

1. Because you feel unwell.
2. Because you feel unattractive.
3. Because you want to live a long healthy life with your family and loved ones.
4. Because you want to glorify God in your body.
5. Because you want to live long enough to fulfill the commission God has placed upon your life.
6. Because when you look at the American population, you decide you do not want to look like them.
7. Because a medical emergency forces you to take action.

I personally had all seven reasons operating in my life. I pray God gives you enough motivation to make the change. I encourage you to get together with friends or family to work through this book and apply it together. Whenever we team up we have more power. Remember, one can put 1000 to flight and two can put 10,000.

Why I Have Decided to Take Responsibility for My Own Health

The Bible says that we can judge by evaluating fruit. My evaluation of the fruit of current medical science and practice was that in certain areas there were great failures. Many degenerative diseases are increasing.

According to their statistics, it is almost guaranteed that cancer would strike my family of four. And the treatments they offer put the person through torture and hell. It just does not seem right. I do not like that fruit. I said, "God must have a better way." So I began to search.

I had assumed that "they" were looking after my health. Once I sat down and thought about who "they" were, I reconsidered my position. "They" were the government, the FDA, the pharmaceutical companies and doctors — of whom many have their own careers and financial interests in mind rather than my health. (Not all doctors arc in this category — just some.)

I had tried Western medicine and it had not helped me with a problem I was facing, so I was kind of thrown out on my own to fend for myself. That, too, helped me take responsibility for my own health.

I challenge you to **take responsibility for your own health.** That is the most basic point I want to get across in this entire book. Do not give away that responsibility. No one cares for your health as much as you do. Western medicine is very limited in its approach to disease at this particular time in history. God has a better plan. Go back to your Bible and find out what God has said. And let your Bible speak to you. Don't relegate it off to a dusty shelf. Let it apply to your life today. It does apply, as thousands of scientific studies have confirmed.

What does it mean to take responsibility for your own health

1. Acquire a general knowledge in the areas of sickness and health. This book is an introduction, and the recommended books are a good follow-up. This will provide a foundation upon which you can continue to build.

2. Gain specific information about any particular problem you are facing. This can be done through talking with doctors, talking with other people, reading books, going to a good library, and subscribing to good prevention and health care newsletters. I suggest tackling the problem with the earnest resolve that you are not going to stop your search until you have found fully effective, non-invasive, natural means to resolve your problem. I believe in most, if not all, cases you can find such solutions if you will search diligently. The Bible instructs us to "ask and keep on asking...seek and keep on seeking." Don't take "no" for an answer. If your first twenty inquiries do not get you satisfactory answers, try another twenty until you find your solution. I think your health and the health of

your loved ones is well worth such efforts. Pursue all natural means available as your first recourse.

3.   Analyze and evaluate, pray, discern, and question deeply what you hear, and continue to question until you get good answers.

4.   Try things out on your own body and **listen to your body's response.** What is it saying to you? (One pastor's wife tried some antioxidants I provided for her and found that a fissure [tear] which she had had in her colon for several years was abruptly healed!)

5.   Do these things over and over again, until you arrive at a level of truth which is effective and meaningful.

For example, I just recently decided to **take personal responsibility for the health care of my lower back.** Since falling twenty feet down a hay-shoot and landing on my feet as a young teenager, I have tended to throw my back out every couple of months, requiring a trip to the chiropractor to have it put back in. My inner attitude for years has been that **my chiropractor is the one responsible** to take care of my lower back pain. This attitude is the opposite of taking personal responsibility for my own health. Now I realize that I am the one responsible for taking care of my lower back pain. My move toward responsibility went like this.

I began by asking my chiropractor if there was anything I could do to help keep my back from going out. He said, "Not really. Just come in for an adjustment every month." Next time in I asked him if there were any exercises I could do to help keep it in good condition. He said that he used to offer a whole assortment of excellent overall exercises, but he discovered that most people didn't stay on them so he has stopped offering them. I asked if he could show me any that would be good for my lower back. He showed me about half a dozen. I was only able to remember two or three by the time I got home because I learn more by careful study and analysis rather than by just "hearing". In addition, I wasn't sure if I was doing the exercises "right" or not. I was not exactly sure what muscles were supposed to be being stretched, and if I did the exercise improperly, it would be worthless or if I could actually hurt myself. I did learn to do "curl-ups" which are mini-sit-ups rather than full sit-ups as I had done all my life. I learned that full sit-ups can much more easily hurt your body. I learned that curl-ups strengthen my stomach muscles which are the "front side of my back" and thus very important to the overall care of my back.

When I was in Florida a year later with my parents, my back acted up. I went to Mom's chiropractor and asked if he could recommend any exercises. He gave me a sheet which pictured and described various exercises for the back. I went home and studied it and began doing several. Still, the sheet did not tell me what muscle groups I was stretching in each exercise and what I was supposed to be careful of and what I was to be feeling and any tips about the right or wrong way to do the exercise, so I still **felt very uncertain** when I did several of the exercises. I sent the page to my chiropractor to get his response. He never got back to me, and I never took the initiative to call him for an answer. You know, the Bible teaches that we are to ask and keep on asking, seek and keep on seeking, knock and keep on knocking, and the door will be opened to us. I have tended to stop knocking too soon in my progress toward truth and left myself in confusion and lack of clarity.

Just recently, a friend of mine named Dean Rhoads taught me a very important process for working on a problem. He sits down at his computer and describes the problem and any ways to resolve it. He then comes back to that problem every week, thinking more about it and recording any more thoughts he has about how to resolve the needs and "opportunities" presented by that problem. I have decided to follow this format from now on and not leave problems in an unanswered state but work on them until they are resolved. My advice to you is that if you ask for an answer and don't get a good one, keep right on asking, seeking, and knocking until you do. By so doing, you will much more quickly reap the fruit of knowledge. People perish for lack of knowledge.

My next step was to mention my back problem to my secretary. She immediately responded that her back goes out exactly the same way. She does a few specific stretching exercises and within one to two days it goes right back in again. This sounded too good to be true. Since my back was out at the time, she showed me the exercises so I could begin trying them. I did them for a week and my body said to me, "Your back is still out." So, frustrated, I went to another chiropractor to help get it back in, as mine had already tried twice in the last week and gotten nowhere (at $28 per appointment). The other doctor got it in place (praise God!), and I noticed something else. While he had me lying on my stomach, he checked several times to see if my feet were even. This showed him when my hip joints were properly in place. He finally got them even and I could feel that my hips had slipped back in place.

That reminded me of the "leg-lengthening" prayers very common-place ten years ago in the charismatic movement. Once, when I was doing a seminar in California, my back was out. A lady commented that she sensed my back was out of place and wanted to know if I wanted her to pray for it. I never turn down prayer, so I told her, "Sure!" She had me sit down, held my feet straight out, and saw that they were uneven. She prayed for them to be made even, and sure enough, I felt something move in my hips. It felt like a chiropractic treatment had been given. She declared that they were even and that any time I needed a chiropractic treatment, I could just have someone pray for me as she had and I would receive a heavenly chiropractic treatment. My back was fixed, so I was thrilled. However, I didn't know anyone in New York with the leg-lengthening ministry, so I just let it go. I suppose I could have asked my wife to try it. You never know. Perhaps, God would just do it through her. The Bible does say that we have not because we ask not. Someday, I am really going to start living the whole Bible in simple, childlike faith. Until then, I will probably have to continue living in a level of misery which is not God's perfect will for my life. I am going to make a decision right now, even as I am writing this. If my back goes out again, I am going to have someone pray for me and see if I can receive another heavenly chiropractic treatment.

As I thought about why the stretching exercises worked for my secretary's back and not mine, I came up with a couple of possibilities. Perhaps her back problem is different from mine and, therefore, responds better. Or maybe, since she does stretching exercises regularly and has for years (and I haven't for twenty years), her back could more easily respond and go back into place on its own with much less pressure. Also, she does the exercises as soon as she feels her back go out. My back had been out for about ten days before she showed me some exercises I could do. So even though my body told me her exercises had not worked on me, my mind and heart were saying, "Don't give up yet. I think we are on a good track here."

So I said to Patti, "Let's go to the mall and see if we can find a good book on stretching exercises." We examined several exercise books, and Patti finally suggested one called *Your Personal Trainer* by Ann Goodsell, which I fell in love with for several reasons. First, Ann appeared to be an excellent trainer, as she had trained at least one Olympic Gold Medalist (Sally Gunnell). This made me think she probably knew what she was doing. Second, the book was a publication of Better Homes and Gardens, a well-respected and well-established organization. The book appeared to have credibility. Next, the Table of Contents showed that she dealt with all three basic categories of exercise: stretching, aerobic, and strength-building. I was just realizing that I needed to gain more understanding of how to integrate all three of these categories into my exercise program. So it piqued my interest.

Most exciting to me was Ann's diagram naming each major muscle and tendon group of the human body. As she presented each exercise throughout the book, not only would she describe each step of the exercise with corresponding full color pictures, but she also listed what set of muscles was being stretched by that particular exercise. I found I could refer back to her diagram, locate the muscle group listed for the exercise, and then as I did the exercise, see if I felt **that muscle group** being stretched. By listening to what my body was saying back, I could now accurately determine that I was doing the exercise properly and was stretching the muscles that needed to be stretched. In addition, for each exercise Ann gave a box with "safety tips" or "personal trainer's tips", which are the cautions she normally gives several times throughout the day as she works with trainees. This was **exactly the information I had been looking for** for more than a year and had not been able to find. I wanted to know that I was doing the exercise right, so that I would not be wasting my time or hurting myself. I decided to study her book carefully and become an expert trainee on exercise. Incidentally, some people are more like my wife, who did not need a book like this. She simply watches a good exercise video, follows the trainer, and gets all the right kinds of exercise. So each of us have our preferred way of learning.

That evening at the mall, we also purchased a book on *Walking for Health*. As I scanned through it, I was drawn to the "stretching exercise" section. It described the Ear-to-Knee stretch, which I described in the earlier chapter on exercise. What caught my attention was the following quote: "This valuable stretch relaxes the quadratus lumborum, in Dr. Norelli's view the most overlooked source of low back pain. The quadratus lies deep beneath the spinal muscles and joins the pelvis to the 12th rib. When tight or tender, it can pull you down or off to one side causing you to shuffle. Or there may be unrelenting pain at the belt level in your low back. Sound familiar?"[1]

Well, it was an exact description of what happens to me. So I read on. "The causes of a whacked-out quadratus are legion. A common one is prolonged sitting, awkward lifting...or a quick stooping movement when your torso is twisted....The ear-to-knee stretch helps relax this troublesome muscle....The more relaxed and flexible these muscles are, the more relaxed and pain-free your walk will be."[2]

Finally I was getting somewhere: An exact description of my problem; An exact exercise to do to loosen the muscles which contribute to the problem. I tried the exercise but my muscle was so tense I was able to only partially complete it. Everyone else in my family tried and was easily able to perform it. This further confirmed to me that my lack of stretching for twenty years was a major contributing factor to my lower back problems. Amazingly, within ten days of practicing, my back had limbered up enough so I, too, could perform the complete exercise. Amazing how just a few stretching exercises can do so much!

I noted in the April 1994 issue of Prevention Magazine that Michael Pollock, Ph.D., Director of the Center for Exercise Science at the University of Florida, found that a simple strength-building session **every one or two weeks** may be enough to maintain significant improvements in strength.[3] In another study, a daily stretching program was shown to decrease back pain in just two weeks.[4] The next comment from Prevention sealed my conviction of what I believed was happening to my body. "Dr. Micheli stresses the importance of stretching the ham-strings (in the back of the thighs). Tight hamstrings can tug at the pelvis and alter the alignment of your back. And remember, you are never too old to improve your flexibility. A study of seniors (average age 72) showed that a ten-week program of stretching 20 to 30 minutes a day performed three times a week produced significant improvements in both back flexion and extension."[5]

Well, it was settled for me. My body has confirmed that the way I am living is wrong. I had a feeling in my spirit that what I was learning about stretching exercises was right. My research, finally, showed me what to do about it. My final step was to experiment on my body and see what it said back to me. I went back to the book *Your Personal Trainer* and began carefully studying and practicing the various back- and leg-stretching and muscle-building exercises. I would study them; then I would do them. After a few days, I would go back to study them again to make sure I was doing them correctly. Sometimes, I miss part of the instructions until I have been doing them for awhile. Then when I go back and re-read them, I see things in the instructions which I had not seen before. I went back and forth several times between practice and the manual, all the time listening to my body to see what it was saying to me. Does it feel better? Do I have less back pain? Am I making fewer trips to the chiropractor? If the answer to these questions is yes then I consider myself on the path toward truth. If the answer is no, then I return to the drawing board once again. "Blessed are they who hunger and thirst for righteousness for they shall be filled" (Matt. 5:6).

I did have to go back to the drawing board once again. My back still would not straighten out, so I tried another chiropractor who had sent an advertisement to our home. He seemed great. He x-rayed my lower back, and the x-ray showed a largely disintegrated disk and a fair size bone spur on one of the lower vertebrae. He said that neither could be healed naturally. I called a friend, Linda Basta, who does foot reflexology and asked what she knew. She suggested a citrus calcium product to remove the bone spur but didn't know much about it. She was going to get me the title of a good book she had read on healing back problems.

Later that morning a call came from Robert Gonzales, a consultant from Nature's Wellness. He had read an article I had written where I mentioned natural health and was seeing if he could interest me in their product line. One of their products was a high-grade calcium supplement, which Linus Pauling (the Nobel Prize winner who worked with vitamin C and cancer) had tested and found to be the best on the market in America. My ears picked up on this "chance encounter" phone call. So often, once one asks a question, the answer appears. It seems to be a spiritual principle, and we need to be aware when it happens. To be perfectly honest, I almost was not open to this one, because when I found that the person on the phone wanted to sell me something, I almost closed my mind and heart to him. But I am glad I didn't. Instead, I asked if he knew if their calcium supplement could remove bone spurs. He transferred me to someone in the company who was an expert on the topic, who said, "Absolutely!" and gave some case histories. She said the bone spurs would be gone in about two weeks. She also gave me additional information on how to fix disintegrated disks naturally through nutritional means. I ordered their product for a one-month try. My chiropractor offered to do free x-rays at the end of the trial, because he, too, is interested to see if this calcium will work.

I have two reasons for taking so much time to tell you this story. First, I believe many people have lower back pain and will benefit from my experiences. Second, I want you to use this story as a **model** for the steps you will take when you make the decision to **TAKE RESPONSIBILITY FOR YOUR OWN HEALTH!** This is the foundational shift I want to take place in your life as a result of your reading this book. If you make this change and do **take responsibility for your own health,** you will begin doing processes similar to the one I have described above. It may take you several months or years to fully research an area and get the answers you need. However, if you write down your problem and work weekly on ideas that can help you solve it, you will find solutions more quickly than if you just take a stab at it every once in awhile when it painfully demands your attention.

My Paradigm for Establishing Truth

It is easy to become confused from reading conflicting reports on various health measures and what to do and how to eat. Let me share with you my system (paradigm) for discovering truth. It is based on six pillars which are listed below.

1. Illumined Scriptures (Luke 24:32)

2. Illumined thoughts in one's mind (Luke 1:3)

3. Illumined witness in one's heart (Mark 2:8)

4. Illumined counsel of others (Prov. 11:14)

5. Illumined understanding of life's experiences — one's fruit (Matt. 7:16)

6. Illumined revelation from God through dreams, visions, prophecy and journaling (Acts 2:17)

As a Christian, I always start by checking the Bible to see what the Holy Spirit will illumine from the Word of God.

The Bible instructs me to check with several other sources also. For example, the Bible says "By their fruit you shall know them" (Matt. 7:16), so I always look at the fruit of a proposed direction. I look at several kinds of fruit. One is the fruit in the person's own life. If he is instructing me on how to live or how to eat, what does he himself look like? Is he strong, slim, vibrant, and healthy? He is the fruit of his counsel. Do I want to look like him ten years from now? I also look at the fruit of others who have followed his way. As a group, am I satisfied with the results I am seeing? If not, then I hold the advice in question. That is precisely why I question the advice of Western medicine at this particular juncture of history. The statistics on the advance of degenerative diseases are alarming. I do not want to be part of the death toll. So I will look elsewhere for counsel.

The Bible also says, "In the multitude of counselors there is safety" (Prov. 11:14). So I check around, especially with those who are producing **good fruit** in the area I am seeking instruction. They will become my most cherished counselors. When I find other cultures of the world eating a different diet and having far less degenerative disease, I examine what they are doing. When I discover that their diet lines up with the first diet that God gave to man, then I start getting excited. I sense revelation could be flowing and about to enlighten me.

I also check with my mind (Luke 1:3). Does what is being said make sense? Can I understand it, especially when I ask God to anoint my reasoning ability and I go with anointed, flowing thoughts? Can I articulate it and prove it with some scientific studies?

I check with my heart. Do I feel peace (Phil. 4:7) or unrest at the deepest level within? I do not mean an unrest in my soul. I mean an unrest or peace on the deeper level, the level of my spirit. And I check with the voice of God within my heart. What do I sense God saying directly to me through dream, vision, intuition, prophecy, and journaling?

I look for all six of the above pillars to line up before I assume I have truth. Then, of course, since the Bible says that we see through a glass darkly, I still may not have truth. However, I am as right as I know to be at this particular point in my life. And that is all I can be. That is what I offer you.

To use the above paradigm, one must be humble, teachable, flexible, open, and changeable. There is a need to be a constant learner, to examine many different streams of thought on an issue, from many different perspectives. I have discovered that many people will not do this, and so, many walk in quite a bit of ignorance, arrogance, and pride. That is truly one of the great misfortunes in life. I pray it will not be yours.

Gaining Knowledge

I decided to study and research the area of health, talk with others, and test things on my own body to see what works for me. It has been a fascinating study. I cannot believe what I have learned, nor how my health and vitality have improved. I am ecstatic and would love for each of you to experience the same.

I have decided that of all the books I read, there are a few which are so basic and foundational that everyone should have them in their library. Most of these books are recommended and described earlier in this book. I will list them again here.

Life Pack!

The key foundational books which everyone should own are:

1. *The McDougall Plan* by John McDougall
2. *McDougall's Medicine: A Challenging Second Opinion* by John McDougall
3. *The McDougall Health Supporting Cookbooks Vol. 1 & 2* by Mary McDougall
4. *The Cancer Answer* by A. E. Carter and Larry Lymphocyte
5. *Counseled by God* by Mark and Patti Virkler
6. *Power Healing* by John Wimber
7. *Fast Your Way to Health* by Lee Bueno
8. *Your Personal Trainer* by Ann Goodsell
9. *Options: The Alternative Cancer Therapy Book* by Richard Walters (see description below)
10. *Prescription for Nutritional Healing* by James & Phyllis Balch
11. *Disease Free* by Matthew Hoffman, William LeGro and the editors of <u>Prevention Magazine</u>

The book *Disease Free* has not been mentioned before. It is a reference book listing more than 150 illnesses and conditions. Natural remedies are discussed, followed by possible surgeries which are also used in treating the problem. It contains advice from over 300 doctors. It is a wonderful bridge between natural approaches and surgical procedures. My personal approach is to try all the methods listed in the book *Eden's Health Plan: Go Natural!*. Then, if I still have a critical unmet need, I will go to Western medicine to help me fix it up. I am largely a pragmatist. I do what works. Western medicine is excellent in healing broken bones and sewing up damaged body parts and performing emergency operations. I respect that ability greatly.

Books numbered 8 - 11 are reference books which you will not necessarily read through, but which you will refer to when specific ailments arise. Also, the cookbooks in number three will not be read through but will be referenced as desired. So only six of the recommended books are ones you will sit down and read through. If you read one book a month, you will cover them in just half a year, and your life will be dramatically improved for the better. You probably cannot make a better health decision than this. I urge you to do so. Applying the information in these books may take you a year but will probably add ten years to your life, save you a $25,000 operation, and provide vibrant health throughout your life. It is well worth your investment!

For additional help in specific areas, read the following:

If you have cancer:
The Cancer Battle Plan by Anne E. Frahm

If you need motivation to exercise:
Walking for Health by Mark Bricklin

If you need more teaching on how to hear God's voice:
Communion With God or *Dialogue With God* by Mark & Patti Virkler

If you need more information about the toxins in household cleaners and personal skin care items:
Why Are You Poisoning Your Family? by Kare Possick

If you want to improve your vision:
Natural Vision Improvement by Janet Goodrich

To overcome Candida:
Candida Elimination Program by Kimberly Bright Cassano
Who Killed Candida? by Vicki Glassburn

To deal with bronchitis and asthma:
Breathe Again Naturally by Bernard Jensen

To learn what foods heal what problems:
The Food Pharmacy by Jean Carper

A book on the recommended reading list above which we have not yet described is *Options: The Alternative Cancer Therapy Book*. *Options* has been written for those seeking a clearer understanding of the alternative therapies used in the treatment of cancer. It covers the full spectrum of available alternative methods, from biologically-based approaches to immune-enhancing treatments, dietary and nutritional regimes, herbal and plant- based remedies, biolectric medicine, and adjunctive therapies. It also includes the latest experimental advances in cancer treatment.

Using plain and simple language, *Options* accurately — and without bias — explains how each treatment works, presents the scientific rationale underlying each method, and provides clinical documentation of the results. The book further examines the myths and misconceptions surrounding alternative cancer therapies from both political and social perspectives. In addition, *Options* provides important guidelines for choosing an alternative treatment, as well as detailed information on referral services that can help you select the therapies best suited to your personal needs. To make an informed decision, it is vital to have access to the right information. *Options* will put that information in your hands when you need it.

The introductory pages of *Options* state the following: "Cancer is this century's Black Plague. At least one in three Americans will develop cancer; of those, roughly two-thirds will die within five years....Another one-half of the remaining patients die between their fifth and tenth years." So to claim a cure, one really needs to wait ten years, not five as is commonly misrepresented. The number of Americans with cancer will double within this decade, making it the nation's leading cause of death, according to MediTrends 1991-1992, a report by the American Hospital Association. (The report can be ordered by calling 800-AHA-2626.) Wouldn't it be amazing if this Black Plague were stopped in the same way as the last one, by Christians reading and applying laws from the Bible on diet, health, and nutrition. I have no doubt this will happen. May you and I be ones who apply the Holy Bible to society's problems and experience God's covenant of health as a result. May we spread the good news to others.

I believe everyone should read *Options*, even if they do not have cancer. Since the cancer epidemic is so large today (and growing), the probability is high that someone you know and love will get cancer, even if you don't. It is a bit late to calmly meditate through a 400-page resource book when you have just been told you or your friend or loved one has cancer and needs invasive treatments immediately. Then you are generally too shattered to think clearly. Let's go through this book while we still have our wits about us.

Let me describe just one of the many services this book puts you in touch with: the "International Association of Cancer Victors and Friends". The service provides an individualized, in-depth report on your specific medical problem, with information from medical texts and journals; lay-oriented newsletters, books, and magazines; and computer databases. The reports range in length from 110 to 150 pages and include the latest information, pro and con, on both orthodox and alternative therapies. They address your individual situation, for example, "Should I take chemotherapy for node-negative breast cancer?" Shorter reports are also available. This is just one of the many services of which this book makes you aware.

Our Reduced Risk of Cancer

By practicing the principles of this book, *Eden's Health Plan: Go Natural!*, you are effectively eliminating 95 percent or more of your chance of getting cancer! The following diagram on cancer risk factors with percentages is taken from the book Everyone's Guide to Cancer Therapy by Dr. Samuel Broder, director of the National Cancer Institute.[6]

Eating the Genesis Diet and some superfoods will eliminate the 35 percent cancer risk caused by diet. Not consuming tobacco removes another 32 percent of risk. The 10 percent risk caused by viruses and infections can be decreased or eliminated through building your im-

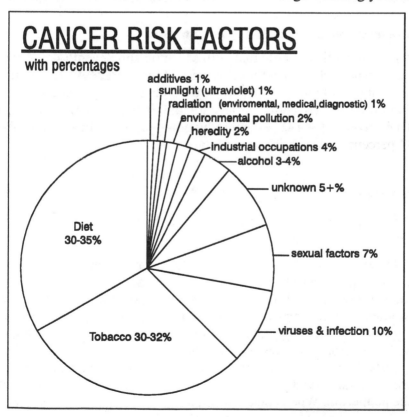

CANCER RISK FACTORS
with percentages

additives 1%
sunlight (ultraviolet) 1%
radiation (enviromental, medical,diagnostic) 1%
environmental pollution 2%
heredity 2%
industrial occupations 4%
alcohol 3-4%

unknown 5+%

Diet
30-35%

sexual factors 7%

viruses & infection 10%

Tobacco 30-32%

mune system with the use of aloe and destroying bacteria with colloidal silver. The seven percent caused by sexual factors (i.e. age of a woman when she first had intercourse and first becomes pregnant and AIDS-related cancers) is overcome by living morally pure lives. The four percent caused by alcohol is eliminated by abstaining from alcohol. The four percent caused by industrial occupations can be overcome by working in a non-toxic situation and using non-toxic household cleaners, soaps, detergents, and skin creams, and taking antioxidants. The two percent caused by environmental pollution can be neutralized by the use of an air purifier and a water filter, and taking antioxidants to remove the damage that occurs when you are in smog-filled cities. The one percent caused by additives can be overcome by abstaining from meats and processed foods, eating organic, and taking antioxidants. The five percent unknown can be taken care of by prayer and maintaining a positive mental attitude. Isn't it refreshing to know you can make such a difference in your own risk of cancer? Let us be living testimonies that God has established a covenant of health with His people!

Mormons and Seventh-day Adventists

It is interesting to note that both Mormon and Seventh-day Adventists men have about half the cancer risk of the average American male.[7] Of course, by looking at the above diagram it is easy to see why. They don't use tobacco, coffee, or alcohol, and they live morally pure lives. That accounts for a 45 percent reduction right there. In addition, about 44 percent of Adventists are vegetarian.[8]

So How Am I living Today?

Each person must determine the way he will live. Following is my current testimony of how I am living.

I have changed to the Genesis diet for the most part. I have dropped about 90 percent of the meats I used to eat, and perhaps 70 percent of the dairy products. I did not find as much harmful data against dairy products as I did against meat, so I was stricter in removing meat from my diet. The two big problems with dairy products are their high fat and the intolerance our systems have to digesting lactose. Yogurt adjusts the lactose, so I switched to low-fat yogurt when I want an ice cream sundae. And you can put low-fat cheese on your pizza and skip the pepperoni. When I do eat meat, it is mostly white meats rather than red. Since I do eat a bit of meat, I take acidophilus in the morning to restore the proper flora in my intestines.

I still have some white sugar and white flour, but I have cut most of it out. For a sweet snack, I eat a healthy chocolate-flavored fiber bar instead of a Snickers bar. There are many low- and no-fat snacks in the store if I have such a craving. I suggest you go for a walk through your local grocery store and discover all the low-fat and non-fat foods there are on the shelves. You will be pleasantly surprised. Pretzels are also a great healthy snack food. And don't forget luscious fresh fruit! My favorite beverage is pure water.

Since I am Type A personality and tend toward higher cholesterol levels, I do three additional things: I eat a cereal called Fiber One (found in the grocery store) which interferes with my body's production of cholesterol, and I also take Cholestrex, a capsule found in health food stores which reduces cholesterol. If you need even more help with high cholesterol levels, take Shak-lee's "Heart Plan" drink. These three things together lowered my cholesterol considerably. Without them, even eating right and exercising did not keep my cholesterol down. Perhaps when God has mellowed a bit more of my Type A responses to life, I shall be able to drop these extras. Perhaps not.

Temper Law with Grace!

I am not under law, but under grace. If I want to splurge and feast, I do so. But then I come back to a low-fat, low-cholesterol, high-fiber diet. I recommend you temper law with grace so you do not bring out rebellion in your children or in yourself. I am changing my diet because I want to, not because I have to. Let's be sure to always motivate rather than drive.

Because we do not eat organic food, I take some excellent natural multi-vitamins, a calcium supplement, and an antioxidant. I also take a DHEA precursor and some herbs as desired. I eat an algae superfood both in capsule form and in a small energy bar.

Because we cook our food and thus destroy the enzymes, I take a couple of enzyme capsules with my meal.

We have a water purifier on our kitchen faucet, as well as a Living Water system for the entire house. And we plan to put a purifier on our shower head to remove the chlorine.

When winter comes we will be installing an air purifier in our home. For now, I keep my windows open to keep the house aired out.

How much extra does it cost me to live this way?

Omitting meats and dairy products produces a savings. Exercising is free, opening my windows is free, and putting a $160 water purifier with a five-year warranty on my kitchen faucet is almost free. Of course, I have by now reduced my doctor bills by over 50 percent for the year (probably by 90 percent), so that is a great savings. The fasting saves money, the colon cleanse which I do with the fast costs a bit so the two together balance out to no cost and no savings. Prayer is free and so are faith, hope, and love.

Now I will take the money I have saved and put it toward the following: multi-vitamins and calcium supplements; herbs and chromium; antioxidants; acidophilus; enzymes; algae; and DHEA precursor. If you have trouble affording any of this, contact me (or the person who gave you this book) and I (or they) will show you a creative way that has covered the cost of all these products for me.

I am taking a fair amount of supplements. I do not see that as a negative, because I live in a time and place of devitalized food and extremely poisonous conditions on every hand. These are critical times, and so they demand critical measures if one does not want to die of the twentieth century black plague. Let us choose a path that will allow us to fulfill God's call and commission upon our lives.

Handling Special Situations

There are some additional products I use when necessary.

When I am fighting infection, I take extra aloe capsules and colloidal silver. (See appendix concerning colloidal silver.) When I have a sore back or some other inflamed part in my body, I take extra pycnogenol. When I get a cut, scratch, poison ivy, or athlete's foot, I use melaleuca products.

God has made our bodies and appetites quite flexible

I am exercising about five times a week. I have included stretching and muscle-building along with aerobic exercises and have switched from jogging to fast walking. I never thought I could make that change, but once I tried it, it wasn't hard at all. Maybe this can be a lesson to us to at least try things for a few weeks to see if we can adjust. I believe the human body is very adaptable. If you ask God to help you and commit yourself to a change, you will find your food cravings changing in just a few short weeks. You can learn to love a healthy lifestyle just as easily as you can learn to love a junk food lifestyle.

I will fast at least once a year, accompanied with the colon cleanse. And I pray for healing regularly, and walk in faith, hope, and love.

Listen to your body

One of the most important things you can do is listen to your body. What is it saying to you? If you will listen and respond, your body will tell you what it wants and what it needs. Because white sugar interferes with its ability to communicate clearly to you, the lower your intake of white sugar, the more accurately your body will be able to respond. For years I didn't listen to my body. Now I try to stay attuned to what it is asking me to eat and do. Your final test is your own body. Become skilled in hearing what it is saying to you.

Listen to God's voice

Learn to honor the intuition that flows within you, the impressions that come to you. Often it is God directing you how to live. Test these impressions with the other five pillars for discovering truth and then act upon them. Once you have put the information on your "hard drive" (brain), then let your "software" (the intuitive voice of your spirit) select the right piece for you to be paying attention to on a day-to-day basis. It is critically important that you learn to live this way. If you need help, read *Communion with God* of *Dialogue with God* by the same authors.

Subscribe to a few good health magazines

There are scores of health magazines on the market. It would probably be wise for all of us to subscribe to one or two, just so we are kept abreast of current findings and research. I personally can recommend two: Prevention Magazine (to subscribe write Prevention, P.O. Box 7305, Red Oak, IA 51591-2305), and Dr. Julian Whitaker's Health & Healing newsletter (to subscribe call 1-800-777-5015). Dr. Whitaker will keep you abreast of natural discoveries in medicine as well as new medical procedures which do not work and you should stay clear from. I cannot recommend Dr. Whitaker's newsletter highly enough. You will find it immensely valuable.

If you are interested in a vegetarian magazine, you might want to subscribe to <u>Vegetarian Times</u> an excellent monthly magazine (1-800-435-9610).

How to find a nutritional doctor

If you want to find a nutritionally-oriented doctor in your area, please call the American College for the Advancement of Medicine at 714-583-7666. Or you can simply send them a self-addressed legal-size envelope with 52 cents postage on it and a request for them to send you a free list of nutritional doctors. Send your request to ACAM, P.O. Box 3427, Laguna Hill, CA. 92652.

Another resource is the National Health Federation, P.O. Box 688, Monrovia CA. 91017. You can call them at 818-357-2181 and ask for names of natural health practitioners in your area. They ask a $10 donation for this service.

A third resource is *Third Opinion: An International Directory to Alternative Therapy Centers for the Treatment and Prevention of Cancer* by John M. Fink, Wayne, NJ: Avery Publishing, Inc., 1988.

Another resource is to begin asking people in your city if they can recommend a good natural doctor. Ask and keep on asking, seek and keep on seeking.... As a result of this study, I changed general practitioners and chiropractors. I looked for doctors who were more natural and took time to instruct me in my own healing. I found I had to visit several doctors before I settled on one whom I was comfortable with. Please take your freedom and do the same, if necessary.

Challenges and Questionnaires

At the close of this book, there are several questionnaires and challenges. The "Quality of Life Questionnaire" has a maximum score of 135 and a mean score of 81. In other words, to maintain your health you need a score of at least 81 points. I took this questionnaire twice, once answering the questions according to the way I was living a year ago, before I began this study on health, and again as I am living today. My first score was 55 points and my score today is 119. So this year has been a very fruitful growth experience in my life. I pray it will prove to be as fruitful in your life.

Standard question before any operation

If ever a doctor wants to operate on you, remember to ask him this question: "Would you please show me a study that proves an increase in life span if I submit to this operation, as opposed to my not being operated on." If he cannot show you one, rethink your options! I did ask my general practitioner this question, since he believed in using mastectomies to lengthen life. He was sure there were such studies. I asked him to please find one and show it to me. So far, he hasn't.

Only the Beginning

This book is only the beginning. Next, you will want to read the books recommended earlier in this chapter, and, perhaps, try out various products mentioned throughout this book to see how your body responds to them. (There is an ordering form at the close of the book.)

In addition, there are many other areas of natural approaches to health that we have not even begun to explore in this book, which you may want to acquaint yourself with as you go along. Life is surely a marvelous journey for those who take the time to enjoy it and explore along the way. You will want to hold up each healing methodology to the six pillars for discovering truth, which we mentioned earlier in this chapter, to make sure it is compatible with Scriptural truth. Feel free to pursue those which do not violate Scriptural truth. A few of those which I sense do not violate any clear biblical teaching or principle include naturopathy, nutritional therapies, homeopathy, foot reflexology, chiropractic, and many, many others.

Team Up

Almost everything is easier when you team up with someone else. Hopefully your whole family will work together to pursue health. Some of you may want to form teams at church, or join a health club for support. Do what you need to do to become effective in this change.

A video and/or cassette series (with a workbook) of Mark Virkler teaching through this book is available. This can be useful for either individual or group use. College credit for this course on natural health is offered through Christian Leadership University. Write to request a free course syllabus detailing complete requirements. Mark is also available to do weekend seminars on this subject (1-716-652-6990).

A Vision Concerning God's Army

I have a vision of a renaissance network of Spirit-filled Christians who take God's voice and creativity into **every area** of life. These believers learn to hear the voice of God, receive His divine creativity, wisdom, and direction on a daily basis, and live it out in the areas God has called them to minister. This vast army of people will minister God's grace and kingdom into **every** area of life. In this book, you see the need for these people to serve as farmers, doctors, health practitioners, nutritionists, medical scientists, government regulatory officials, researchers and many other vocations/positions.

Because Spirit-led believers have not led in these vocations in recent years, these areas have gone way offtrack, bringing incredible damage, pain, and death to many people's lives. I pray that you will agree that because the earth is the Lord's (Ps. 24:1), **all areas of life are to be considered ministry,** and you will become a full-time minister in whatever area God is calling you.

As you do, the Church will once again live the covenant blessings which God gave to His children in Deuteronomy 28:1-14. God's children will once again become the head and not the tail, they will be above and not underneath, and they will lend and not borrow. We desperately need men and women demonstrating God's divine revelation in every area of life. Perhaps you will become one of them.

With such godly leadership, hopefully we will live in good health **long enough** to accomplish God's vision of leadership for our own lives. It seems that it takes most of us at least forty years to acquire enough wisdom and understanding to begin to press into leadership roles. What a terrible time for a heart attack or the beginnings of poor health to strike!

The Challenge

So I challenge doctors, farmers, nutritionists, researchers, and government regulators to become part of God's renaissance network. I challenge you to learn to hear the voice of God and to apply it to the ministry you have here in this world. I challenge you to learn to work **with** the laws of nature, not against them. I challenge you to be willing to lay down your life for the truth you discover, realizing that as you lose your life, you gain it. This will require many to step out of the pattern of the world around them. The world of health and farming and government in **America is off track**. It needs reformers to restore it. I have chosen to be one of those reformers. I pray you will be one, also, so the world can be a better place.

Needed: A Renaissance Army

Today God is calling for an army of men and women who will give up their lives to become part of a renaissance army that will restore every area of society. We had hoped that our doctors had studied health. Instead, they have studied pathology (sickness). Now, we must study health. We had hoped that our pastors had studied the ways of the Holy Spirit. Instead, they have studied Biblical law. Now, we must study the ways of the Holy Spirit. We had hoped that our elected officials would be statesmen and public servants. Instead, they are politicians and rule with deception. Now, we must become statesmen. We had hoped that our businessmen would give their lives to serve their employees and customers. Instead, they served their own financial ends. Now, we must demonstrate servanthood in the business world.

God is looking for an army that will take up these and many similar positions. He is asking for you and me to join and take our rightful places in this mighty overcoming army. I will take mine. Will you? Will you lead in the areas God is asking you to lead? Will you seek out God's voice and His principles (as recorded in the Holy Bible) in that area, bringing restoration, renaissance, and rebirth to that area? I pray you will. Perhaps we can take the next year to focus on health and become professionals in the ways of health. Then we can go on from there.

Additional Resources

Trinity School of Natural Health 401 Kings Highway, Winona Lake, IN 46590 is a correspondence school "committed to a holistic understanding of man which is taught in the Scriptures. A healthy or whole person is one who enjoys a balanced life mentally, physically and spiritually. The school makes no apology for faith assumptions concerning the creation of man, the nature of man, the resurrection, eternity or any other subject which does not lend itself to double-blind studies, scientific duplication or investigation." They offer a Master Herbalist Program and a Doctor of Naturopathy Program. (1-800-428-0408.)

Clayton School of Natural Medicine (a correspondence school through which you can earn various degrees — Bachelors, Masters Doctorates — i.e. Masters in Herbology, Masters in Natural Medicine).

Write for their catalog at 2140 11th Ave South Suite 305, Birmingham AL 35205-2841. Phone 205-933-2215.

Help us write our follow-up book — *Go Natural! - Testimonies of Healing*

We are hoping to write a follow-up book which will be full of your stories of how you implemented the principles of this book and restored your health. It should be an exhilarating confirmation that the Bible contains the answers to today's black plagues. We would love you to send us your testimony. Please send the completed form, "I Took the 30-Day Challenge" along with any additional information which makes your story more complete. Become part of the solution, and let your life's testimony inspire others to come back to the Word of God.

References

[1] Bricklin, Mark and Maggie Spilner, *Walking for Health* (Emmaus, PA: Rodale Press, 1992), pp. 174, 175.

[2] Bricklin, p. 175.

[3] Schwade, Steve, "Get Your Back on Track," Prevention Magazine, volume 46, number 4 (April 1994), p. 68.

[4] Spine, March 1992, as cited by Schwade, p. 69.

[5] Journal of Sports Medicine & Physical Fitness, 1991, as cited by Schwade, p. 69.

[6] Dollinger, Malin, Ernest Rosenbaum and Greg Cable, *Everyone's Guide to Cancer Therapy* (Kansas City, MO: Andrews and McMeel, 1991), from the Preface by Dr. Samuel Broder, director of the National Cancer Institute, p. 6.

[7] Padus, Emrika, *Your Emotions and Your Health* (Emmaus, PA: Rodale Press, 1986), p. 82.

[8] Padus, p. 83.

Appendix A

How Can I Get Closer to God?

You may be wanting to improve your relationship with God. Or, you may want to be sure that you will go to heaven when you die. You may have enjoyed the journaling which Mark did in Chapter Ten of this book and long to be able to have the same kind of experience in your own life. The wonderful thing is, you can! Here's how.

The Bible teaches that God hungers to share His love with you. In the Garden of Eden, God walked and talked with Adam and Eve in the cool of the day. That is what God wants to do with each of us, also. He yearns to be able to share His love with us and have us share our hearts with Him on a daily basis. As our Creator and Sustainer, He knows what we need even more than we do, and He answers our questions even before we ask.

God's heart was broken when sin entered into Adam and Eve's lives and stole away that relationship He had with them. The tempter tempted Adam and Eve to live like gods themselves, rather than enjoy the flow of God's life through them. In choosing to look to self, rather than looking beyond to the wonderful Giver of Life, Adam and Eve cut off much of the flow of God within them.

So God sent His Son, Jesus of Nazareth, in the form of a man, to remove the sin which separated mankind's heart from the heart of God. By entering the world as a man, God was able to take the sins of the entire world upon His own shoulders and pay the penalty of this separation by allowing His Son Jesus Christ to be separated from Him for a moment of time. That is why Jesus cried out while dying on the cross, "My God, My God, why have You forsaken Me?" However, in forsaking His Son for a moment of time, God was restoring the opportunity for you and me to return to the experience of the Garden of Eden and, once again, have fellowship with Almighty God. Once again, we could walk with Him in the cool of the day and share our lives with Him and have God share His life with us.

So our relationship with God can be enhanced. We can be sure of going to heaven by receiving the sacrifice of Jesus' life for our sins. The steps are quite clearly laid out in the Bible. They are as follows:

1. **Acknowledge:** "For all have sinned, and fall short of the glory of God" (Romans 3:23).
2. **Repent:** "Repent, then, and turn to God, so that your sins may be wiped out..." (Acts 3:19).
3. **Confess:** "If you confess with your mouth, 'Jesus is Lord,' and believe in your heart that God raised Him from the dead, you will be saved" (Romans 10:9).
4. **Forsake:** "Let the wicked forsake his way and the evil man his thoughts. Let him turn to the Lord...for He will freely pardon" (Isaiah 55:7).
5. **Believe:** "For God so loved the world that He gave His one and only Son, that whoever believes in Him shall not perish but have eternal life" (John 3:16).
6. **Receive:** "He came to that which was His own, but His own did not receive Him. Yet to all who received Him, to those who believed in His name, He gave the right to become children of God" (John 1:11,12).
7. **Spirit:** "If the Spirit of Him who raised Jesus from the dead dwells in you, He who raised Christ Jesus from the dead will also give life to your mortal bodies through His Spirit who indwells you" (Romans 8:11).

A Prayer of Response

If you want a closer relationship with God, if you want to know for certain that when you die you will go to heaven, then offer the following prayer to God, from the depths of your heart. Pray aloud.

"Precious Holy Spirit, do a work in my heart as I offer the following prayer to God.

"God, I come to you in the name of your Son, the Lord Jesus Christ. I acknowledge that I have sinned and fallen short of Your ways. I repent of my sin and ask that the blood of Jesus Christ cleanse me of all my sins. I receive this cleansing even now as You sweep over my soul. I confess with my mouth that Jesus Christ is the Son of God and the Lord of my life. I invite You, Jesus, to have first place in my heart and my life. I believe God raised Jesus from the dead, and that He is alive in my heart today. I forsake any evil ways and thoughts which I have harbored and this day turn my life over to Jesus. I ask, Jesus, that You fill my heart and my mind with Your ways and Your thoughts and that You begin a transforming work from within my heart and my spirit. By bclicving in Jesus and His life within me, I am assured a place in heaven with God. I receive eternal life this day. Thank you, Lord Jesus Christ. I yield myself right now to the movings of the Holy Spirit within my spirit. Holy Spirit, please make this very real in my heart and let me sense your movings within me. May you seal this prayer this day."

Now just wait quietly for a few minutes in the presence of God and His Holy Spirit and see what you sense within. Lift up your eyes to Jesus and humbly receive His life within your soul.

Record below any impressions or sensations which you received in your heart and soul as you prayed this prayer.

Date I prayed this prayer: _____

Assurance: "But these are written that you may believe that Jesus is the Christ, the Son of God, and that believing you may have life in His name" (John 20:31).

If you have just prayed the above prayer, we invite you to write or call for a free book giving you an even deeper understanding of your salvation experience. Contact us at Communion With God Ministries, 1431 Bullis Road, Elma, N.Y. 14059. (800) 466-6961.

We also have a series of follow-up courses utilizing books, cassettes, and videos which will train you in many spiritual areas and equip you for greater effectiveness in all of life. These study materials can be used in independent study or as an external degree student of Christian Leadership University, a university which leads to Bachelors, Masters, and Doctoral degrees.

We love you and do want to hear from you if you have just prayed to receive Christ, so do contact us.

Yours in Christ,
Mark & Patti Virkler

——————— RESPONSE FORM ———————

Name _____ Phone _____

Address _____

City_____ State _____ Zip _____

I prayed to accept Jesus Christ as my Lord and Savior on the following date _____.

Check the following which apply:

_____ Please send me additional free information helping me understand and deepen my new life in Jesus.

_____ Please send me free information on additional courses which I may take through Christian Leadership University which will help strengthen my life.

_____ Please send me information on how to find a good group of like-minded believers in my area with whom I can fellowship and relate.

Appendix B

You Can Hear
God's Voice

The age in which we live is so married to rationalism and cognitive, analytical thought that we almost mock when we hear of one actually claiming to be able to hear the voice of God. However, we do not mock for several reasons. First, men and women throughout the Bible heard God's voice. Also, there are some highly effective and reputable men and women of God alive today who demonstrate that they hear God's voice. Finally, there is a deep hunger within us all to commune with God and hear Him speak within our hearts.

As a Bible-believing, born-again Christian, I struggled unsuccessfully for years to hear God's voice. I prayed, fasted, studied my Bible, and listened for a voice within, all to no avail. **There was no inner voice that I could hear!** Then God set me aside for a year to study, read, and experiment in the area of learning to hear God's voice. During that time God taught me **four keys that opened the door to two-way prayer.** I have discovered that not only do they work for me but they have worked for many thousands of Christians who have been taught to use them, bringing tremendous intimacy to their Christian experience and transforming their very way of living. This will happen to you also as you seek God, utilizing the following four keys. They are all found in Habakkuk 2:1,2. I encourage you to read this passage before going on.

Key # 1 — God's voice in our hearts sounds like a flow of spontaneous thoughts. Therefore, when I tune to God, I tune to spontaneity.

The Bible says, "the Lord answered me and said..."(Hab. 2:2). Therefore, Habakkuk knew the sound of God's voice. The Bible describes it as a still, small voice. I guess I had always listened for an inner **audible** voice, and surely God can and does speak that way at times. However, I have found that for most of us, most of the time, God's inner voice comes to us as **spontaneous thoughts, visions, feelings, or impressions.** For example, haven't each of us had the experience of driving down the road and having **a thought come to us** to pray for a certain person? We generally acknowledge this as the voice of God speaking to us to pray for that individual. My question to you is, "What did God's voice sound like as you drove in your car? Was it an inner, audible voice, or was it a spontaneous thought that lit upon your mind?" Most of you would say that God's voice came to you as a spontaneous thought.

So I thought to myself, maybe when I listen for God's voice, I should be listening for a flow of spontaneous thoughts. Maybe spirit-level communication is received as spontaneous thoughts, impressions, feelings, and visions. Through experimentation and feedback from thousands of others, I am now convinced that this is so.

The Bible confirms this in many ways. The definition of *paga*, the Hebrew word for intercession, is "a chance encounter or an accidental intersecting". Therefore, as God lays people on our hearts for intercession, He does it through *paga*, a chance encounter thought accidentally intersecting our thought processes. Therefore, when I tune to God, I tune to chance encounter thoughts or spontaneous thoughts. When I am poised quietly before God in prayer, I have found that the flow of spontaneous thoughts that comes is quite definitely from God.

Key # 2 — I must learn to still my own thoughts and emotions, so that I can sense God's flow of thoughts and emotions within me.

Habakkuk said, "I will stand on my guard post and station myself on the rampart..." (Hab. 2:1). Habakkuk knew that in order to hear God's quiet, inner, spontaneous thoughts, he had to first of all go to a quiet place and still his own thoughts and emotions. Psalm 46:10 encourages us to "Be still, and know that I am God." There is a deep inner knowing (spontaneous flow) in our spirit that each of us can experience when we quiet our flesh and our minds.

I have found several simple ways to quiet myself, so that I can more readily pick up God's spontaneous flow. Loving God through a quiet worship song is a most effective means for many (note 2 Kings 3:15). It is as I become still (thoughts, will, and emotions) and am poised before God that the divine flow is realized. Therefore, after I worship quietly and then become still, I open myself for that spontaneous flow. If thoughts come to me of things I have forgotten to do, I write them down and then dismiss them. If thoughts of guilt or unworthiness come to my mind, I repent thoroughly, receive the washing of the blood of the Lamb, and put on His robe of righteousness, seeing myself spotless before the presence of God.

As I fix my gaze upon Jesus (Heb. 12:2), becoming quiet in His presence, and sharing with Him what is on my heart, I find that two-way dialogue begins to flow. Spontaneous thoughts flow from the throne of God to me, and I find that I am actually conversing with the King of Kings.

It is very important that you become still and properly focused if you are going to receive the pure word of God. If you are not still, you will simply be receiving your own thoughts. If you are not properly focused on Jesus, you will receive an impure flow because the intuitive flow comes out of that upon which you have fixed your eyes. Therefore, if you fix your eyes upon Jesus, the intuitive flow comes from Jesus. If you fix your gaze upon some desire of your heart, the intuitive flow comes out of that desire of your heart. To have a pure flow you must first of all become still, and secondly, you must carefully fix your eyes upon Jesus. Again I will say, this is quite easily accomplished by quietly worshiping the King, and then receiving out of the stillness that follows.

Key # 3 — As I pray, I fix the eyes of my heart upon Jesus, seeing in the spirit the dreams and visions of Almighty God.

We have already alluded to this principle in the previous paragraphs; however, we need to develop it a bit further. Habakkuk said, "I will keep watch to see", and God said, "Record the vision" (Hab. 2:1,2). It is very interesting that Habakkuk was going to actually start looking for vision as he prayed. He was going to open the eyes of his heart and look into the spirit world to see what God wanted to show him. This is an intriguing idea.

I had never thought of opening the eyes of my heart and looking for vision. However, the more I thought of it, the more I realized this was exactly what God intends me to do. He gave me eyes in my heart. They are to be used to see in the spirit world the vision and movement of Almighty God. I believe there is an active spirit world functioning all around me. This world is full of angels, demons, the Holy Spirit, the omnipresent God, and His omnipresent Son, Jesus. There is no reason for me not to see it, other than my rational culture, which tells me not to believe it is even there and provides no instructions on how to become open to seeing this spirit world.

The most obvious prerequisite to seeing is that we need to look. Daniel was seeing a vision in his mind and he said, "I was looking....I kept looking....I kept looking" (Dan. 7:1,9,13). Now as I pray, I look for Jesus present with me, and I watch Him as He speaks to me, doing and saying the things that are on His heart. Many Christians will find that if they will only look, they will see. Jesus is Emmanuel, God with us. It is as simple as that. You will see a spontaneous inner vision, in a similar manner to the ways you receive spontaneous inner thoughts. You can see Christ present with you in a comfortable setting, because Christ is present with you in a comfortable setting. Actually, you will discover that inner vision comes so easily you will have a tendency to reject it, thinking that it is just you. (Doubt is satan's most effective weapon against the Church.) However, if you will persist in recording these visions, your doubt will soon be overcome by faith, as you recognize that the content of them could only be birthed in Almighty God.

God continually revealed Himself to His covenant people using dream and vision. He did so from Genesis to Revelation and said that, since the Holy Spirit was poured out in Acts 2:1-4, we should expect to receive a continuing flow of dreams and visions (Acts 2:17, 18). Jesus, our perfect example, demonstrated this ability of living out of ongoing contact with Almighty God. He said that He did nothing on His own initiative, but only that which he **saw the Father doing, and heard the Father saying** (John 5:19,20,30). What an incredible way to live!

Is it actually possible for us to live out of the divine initiative as Jesus did? A major purpose of Jesus' death and resurrection was that the veil was torn from top to bottom, giving us access into the immediate presence of God, and we are commanded to draw near (Heb. 10:19-22). Therefore, even though what I am describing seems a bit unusual to a rational twentieth century culture, it is demonstrated and described as being a central biblical teaching and experience. It is time to restore to the Church what belongs to the Church.

Because of their intense rational nature and existence in an overly rational culture, some will need more assistance and understanding of these truths before they can move into them. They will find this help in the book Communion With God by the same author.

Key # 4 — Journaling, the writing out of our prayers and God's answers, provides a great new freedom in hearing God's voice.

God told Habakkuk to record the vision and inscribe it on tablets...(Hab. 2:2). It had never crossed my mind to write out my prayers and God's answers as Habakkuk did. Actually, this was commanded by God. If you begin to search Scripture for this idea, you will find hundreds of chapters demonstrating it (Psalms, many of the prophets, Revelation). Why, then, had I never thought of it? Why had I never heard a sermon on it?

I decided to call the process journaling, and I began experimenting with it. I discovered it was a fabulous facilitator to clearly discern God's inner, spontaneous flow because as I journaled I was able **to write in faith for long periods of time,** simply believing it was God. I did not have to test it as I was receiving it, (which jams one's receiver), because I knew that when the flow was over I could go back and test and examine it carefully **at that time,** making sure that it lined up with Scripture.

You will be amazed as you attempt journaling. Doubt may hinder you at first, but throw it off, reminding yourself that it is a Biblical concept, and that God is present, speaking to His children. Don't take yourself too seriously. When you do, you become tense and get in the way of the Holy Spirit's movement. It is when we cease **our labors** and enter His rest that God is free to flow (Heb. 4:10). Therefore, put a smile on your face, sit back comfortably, get out your pen and paper, and turn your attention toward God in praise and worship, seeking His face. As you write out your question to God and become still, fixing your gaze on Jesus, who is present with you, you will suddenly have a very good thought in response to your question. Don't doubt it, simply write it down. Later as you go over your journaling, you, too, will be amazed to discover that you are indeed dialoguing with God.

Some final notes. The safeguards which you should establish as you journal are as follows: 1) You should have received Jesus Christ as your personal Lord and Savior (see Appendix A); 2) You should read through at least the New Testament (preferably, the entire Bible); and 3) You should be submitted to solid, spiritual people who can provide covering for your journaling. Finally, all major directional moves which come through journaling should be submitted to the other five pillars used in establishing truth before being acted upon. These were discussed in the last chapter of this book.

Appendix C

Aloe Vera Test Results From Triputic

by Lee Ritter

Mucopolysaccharides (MEOH) Milligrams Per Liter

Product Name	Date of Test	Mucopoly-saccharide Count	Actual Cost to receive 1200mg. MEOH
Kaire Aloe Vera Juice Aloe Gel Beverage 10x Whole Leaf Concentrate	5/16/93	13,840 Mg/L	$2.57
Lametco - Whole Leaf Aloe Concentrate	11/23/92	12,202 Mg/L	$3.14
Aloe - Ace	4/16/92	7,840 Mg/L	$32.06
Diamite - Vitality Aloe Vera Plus	4/16/92	1,960 Mg/L	$11.91
Coat's- Aloe Vera Gel Drink	9/25/91 12/11/91 2/8/92	2,220 Mg/L 520 Mg/L 6,940 Mg/L	$6.99 $29.86 $2.24
Oriana Tru Gel Aloe Vera Juice	2/8/92	3,390 Mg/L 1,240 Mg/L	$3.19 $8.71
Aloeplus	7/31/92	610 Mg/L	$ N/A

Product Name	Date of Test	Mucopoly-saccharide Count	Actual Cost to receive 1200mg. MEOH
George's "Always Active" Aloe Vera	5/1/92	0 Mg/L	$ N/A
Aloe Gold - AIM Corp.	9/26/92	13,980 Mg/L	$9.93
Jason Winters' Finest	10/20/92	590 Mg/L	$8.20
Forever Living	10/1/92	1,960 Mg/L	$7.07
Nature's Sunshine	10/23/92	290 Mg/L	$45.39
Natural High Aloe	10/26/92	40 Mg/L	$364.64
Multiway Aloe Gel	10/23/92	1,230 Mg/L	$6.45
Aloe Farms	1/8/93	570 Mg/L	$6.83
Sunrider Aloe Vera Juice	2/9/93	60 Mg/L	$178.54
Aloe-Maxx Whole Leaf Concentrate	1/27/93	10,360 Mg/L	$8.50

Good aloe vera concentrate can be used internally or externally. The following is a simple summary of the more popular applications of aloe vera.

Internal:

oral ulcers

colitis

dysentery

cancer prevention

heartburn

arthritis/gout

sore throat

halitosis

hemorrhoids/bleeding piles

asthma (breathing vapors)

peptic ulcers

constipation

kidney infection

energy

dropsy

detoxification

mild laxative

indigestion

immune system enhancement

inflamatory bowel disease

External:

blistering
cold burn, frostbite
softening
scar removal
scalds
fistulas
liver spots
acne, blemishes
exzema
optical flash burns
abrasions, bruises
warts
infections: bacterial
skin ulcers and lesions
mouth and gum disease
hair loss, scalp ailments

wind burn
moisturizing
soothing
sunburn
seborrheapsoriasis
viral, fungal
varicose veins
allergic conditions
radiation burn
wounds, cuts
pain, itching, urticaria
welts
skin cancer
animal stings and bites
heat burns of all kinds

Appendix D

Colloidal Silver —
Nature's Antibiotic

Background Research and Documentation

Silver is a powerful natural antibiotic, used for thousands of years, and no known side effects have ever occurred. It acts as a catalyst, disabling the enzymes that disease-causing organisms need to breathe. It is known to kill over 650 of these organisms in six minutes or less, upon contact inside the body. Resistant strains fail to develop, and the body doesn't develop a tolerance. Colloidal silver is both a preventive and a remedy for colds and influenza and all organism-caused diseases. Colloidal silver, pronounced co-loyd-al, is totally safe, effective, and non-toxic.

All living things exist in the colloidal state. Before any medication can be used, the body must convert it from a crystalline state to a colloidal state. Taking colloidal silver orally each day is very much like having a second immune system. This lessens the load on the first immune system, resulting in more vitality. In addition, the toxicity due to the average amount of germinal, viral, and fungal activity naturally occurring in the body is less, resulting in yet greater vigor. You feel much better, more energetic, and more relaxed.

Dr. Robert Becker, while analyzing hair samples, and questioning the parties involved, noticed a correlation between low silver levels and sickness. People who had low silver levels were frequently sick, had innumerable colds, flu, fevers, and other illnesses. He found no silver supplements marketed at that time. He said he believed a silver deficiency was the reason for the improper functioning of the immune system. The presence of silver is also critical to the destruction of bacteria and viruses. Dr. Becker's experiments concluded that silver works on a wide range of bacteria, without any side effects, and without damage to the cells of the body.[1]

Dr. Becker also stated that the silver ion (colloidal state) was doing something more than killing disease-causing organisms. It was also causing major growth stimulation of injured tissues. Human fibroblast cells, common throughout the body, when exposed to silver, differentiated, that is, they changed to an embryonic, general cell able to multiply at a great rate and then differentiate into the specialized cells of the organ or tissue that has been injured, even in patients over fifty years of age. Tissues heal as easily as a child's. Dr. Becker also stated that in the presence of the silver ion, cancer cells change back to normal cells, regardless of their location in the body. He concluded that the presence of the silver ion will regenerate tissue, eliminate old or cancerous cells, and any other diseased or abnormal condition. Two very bad burn cases he studied, having higher than average levels of the silver ion present on the body tissues, were able to quickly regenerate the burn-damaged tissue, without the occurrence of scar tissue or overload of the immune system.

Dr. Becker also stated that the ionic-colloidal form of silver has several other advantages over all other forms, there being no ions other than the silver ion to burden the body tissues or immune system. Moreover, it is especially well suited for use against many types of disease-causing organisms simultaneously, even antibiotic-resistant strains, and fungus. Fantastic successes have been recorded in cases that were considered hopeless. Residual silver in the body more than doubles the killing power of the immune system to destroy cancer cells and other disease-causing organisms.

Dr. Bjorn Nordenstrom, of Sweden, uses silver in his cancer-cure method. He states that the whole thing is so simple he hadn't seen it at first. Even advanced cases have been successfully treated.

Tests prove that due to the high absorption of silver in the small intestine, the friendly bacteria in the large intestine are not affected. Silver aids the developing fetus in growth, health, and eases the delivery and recovery. Based on laboratory tests, all bacteria, viruses, and fungal organisms are killed within six minutes of contact. The more silver in the body, the faster and more frequent the contact will occur.

There is no known disease-causing organism that can live in the presence of even minute traces of the chemical element of simple metallic silver. They are killed in a few minutes or less. There are no side effects. You cannot overdose. It is not wasted if you take fifty times the recommended amount, as it will accumulate in the body to continue the benefit further into the future. The accepted method is to consume a four-ounce bottle monthly in any convenient increments, anytime during the month.

A recent breakthrough in the method of production brings the cost down and the availability up so everyone can enjoy good health.

Colloidal Silver — The Universal Antibiotic

Colloidal silver is considered to be the most universal antibiotic substance that for all practical purposes is non-toxic in its micro-concentration of 3-5 ppm. It has been proven to be useful against over 650 different infectious conditions. Many forms of bacteria, viruses and fungus utilize a specific enzyme for their metabolism. Silver acts as a catalyst, effectively disabling the enzyme. It is toxic to all tested species of fungi, bacteria, protozoa, parasites, and many viruses.

Colloidal silver can be applied directly to delicate mucous membranes, such as those in the eye, with no irritation and with beneficial results....The colloidal particles diffuse gradually throughout the blood and give prolonged therapeutic action.

The highest quality colloidal silver is procured by the electrocolloidal/ non-chemical method, meaning the silver particles and water have been completely "colloided" — simultaneously dispersed within and bound to each other by an electrical current sent through the combination. This process is the only known method to create a truly homogeneous (evenly distributed) suspension. The grade of silver used is also very important.

Colloidal is a substance not water soluble but suspended in liquid form (suspended through a unique electrical process in water).

Silver is taken and precipitated into a liquid medium and held in electrical suspension. As a result, you have a solution that, when consumed, is immediately absorbed and distributed throughout the system. You have is a broad spectrum, non-toxic substance.

Trace minerals in our body allow the body to conduct electricity, and this generates antibiotic functions in the body. Each mineral has a different weight, different level of conductivity, and different frequency. Silver will only irritate single-cell organisms, so it is non-toxic to our bodies.

Colloidal silver is tasteless. You can do anything except cook with it. The amount of silver consumed is very low, but there is no known toxicity level for colloidal silver if it is prepared properly.

In India, silver is used to keep milk fresh and is said to be more effective than pasteurization. Also, a silver coin is put on wounds to fight infection.

Prior to 1938, colloidal silver was considered to be one of the mainstays of antibiotic treatment. At that time it was considered to be quite "high-tech", but compared to today's colloidal silver solutions it was technically inferior. It was administered in just about every way that modern drugs are administered: It was injected both intravenously and intramuscularly, used as a gargle for throat conditions, used as a douche, taken orally, applied topically even on sensitive tissues, and dropped into the eyes and ears.

The comeback of silver in medicine began in the 1970's. The late Dr. Carl Moyer, chairman of Washington University's Department of Surgery, received a grant to develop better treatments for burn victims. Dr. Margraf, as the chief bio-chemist, worked with Dr. Moyer and other surgeons to find an antiseptic strong enough, yet safe to use over large areas of the body. Dr. Margraf reviewed twenty-two antiseptic compounds and found drawbacks in all of them.

"Popular antiseptics...can be used over small areas only." Furthermore, disease organisms can become resistant to antibiotics, triggering a dangerous super-infection. "These compounds are also ineffective against a number of harmful bacteria, including the biggest killer in burn cases — a greenish-blue bacterium called *Pseudomonas acruginosa*. It almost always shows up in burns, releasing a poison."

When the silver nitrate was diluted to a .5 percent solution, they found that it killed the *Pseudomonas acruginosa* bacteria and permitted wounds to heal. Resistant strains did not appear.

Dr. Harry Margraf concluded: Silver is the best all around germ-fighter we have.

In 1919, after describing silver and other metal colloids, Alfred Searle wrote, "The germicidal action of certain metals in the colloidal state having been demonstrated, it only remained to apply them to the human subject, and this has been done in a large number of cases with astonishingly successful results....Fortunately, the recognition of bacteria and their products as essentially colloidal in character has greatly facilitated the study of disinfection. It is now realized that — disregarding the fact that bacteria are alive — they may — owing to their colloidal character — and that of the toxins and some other substances they produce — be destroyed by substances which bear an electrical charge opposite to that of the bacteria or their colloidal products."

C.E.A. MacLeod reports colloidal silver being used with marked success in the following cases:

> "Septic and follicular tonsillitis, Vincent's angina, phlyctenular conjunctivitis, gonorrhoeal conjunctivitis, spring catarrh, impetigo (contagious acne of face and body), septic ulcers of legs, ringworm of body, tinea versicolor, soft sores, supporative appendicitis after operation (the wounds cleaned rapidly), pustular eczema of scalp and pubes, chronic eczema of meatus of ear with recurrent boils, and also chronic eczema of anterior nares, offensive discharge in case of chronic supporation in otitis media, bromidrosis of feet, axillae and blind boils of neck. By infection: Gonorrhoea and chronic cystitis (local), boils, epiditymitis."

Sir James Cantlie found it very effective "in cases of spure, dysentery, and intestinal troubles. Being non-toxic, the dose can be increased from 1 to 2 or more drams (drams = .125 ounces) twice or thrice daily."

A. Legge Roe regarded "stable colloidal silver as a most useful preparation in ophthalmic practice, and particularly in cases of gonorrhoeal ophthalmic, purulent ophthalmic of infants, infected ulcers of the cornea and hypopyon ulcer (tapping of the interior chamber and cautery, and other operative procedures being now rarely required, when if perforation does occur it is smaller and more manageable), interstitial keratitis, blepharitis, dacryocystitis, and burns and other wounds of the cornea. According to this authority, if the great chemosis which usually accompanies the use of silver were adopted in every case of purulent ophthalmia of infants 'there would be no such thing as impaired sight or blindness from this cause.' He has had many cases of interstitial Keratitis in adults, in which the complete opacity of the cornea has become absolutely clear in from three to five months, and anyone who has had much experience of this disease in adults knows how often permanent impairment of sight results, and how long the treatment used to last especially if irritants had been used prior to colloidal treatment...the colloidal sol is dropped in three times a day, the eye being kept closed afterwards for five minutes."

Larry C. Ford, M.D. of the Department of Obstetrics and Gynecology, UCLA School of Medicine — Center for the Health Sciences reported in a letter dated November 1, 1988: "I tested them (the silver solutions) using standard anti-microbial tests for disinfectants. The silver solutions were anti-bacterial for concentrations of 10 5 organisms per ml. of Streptococcus Pyogenes, Staphylococcus Aureus, Neisseria Gonorrhea, Gardnerella Vaginalis, Salmonella Typhi, and other enteric pathogens, and fungicidal for Candida Albicans, Candida Globata, and M. Furfur."

In 1939, Robert J. Hartman write, "Aqueous metallic silver suspensions...are used extensively as a gargle and, in genito-urinary diseases, as a douche, or irrigant for inflamed mucous membranes. Certain of these colloidal suspensions are prepared that can be injected intravenously or intramuscularly."

Jim Powell reported in a Science Digest Article, March 1978 titled "Our Mightiest Germ Fighter", "Thanks to eye-opening research, silver is emerging as a wonder of modern medicine. An antibiotic kills perhaps a half-dozen different disease organisms, but silver kills some 650. Resistant strains fail to develop. Moreover, silver is virtually non-toxic."

There has been extensive research in the use of silver for bone reconstruction. Research into the curative properties of silver has been conducted for many years at the Upstate Medical Center, Syracuse University, Syracuse, NY under the direction of Dr. Robert O. Becker, M.D. (now retired), and Dr. Joseph A. Spadaro. They discovered that silver ions, driven by only microamperes of current, substantially promote bone growth. They were successful in promoting rapid bone growth in cases where bone had not healed for a long period of time (an average of two years). With silver-ion treatment, the bones were rapidly reconstructed. Dr. Becker assumes that silver promotes bone growth because it irritates the body into growing new bone.

Two benefits are realized with the use of silver ions for bone healing: (1) The process is safe. There are no side effects with silver. (2) Silver being bactericidal, it sanitizes that area allowing the body to replace bone cells without any of the restraining effects of bacteria.

Becker, R., M.D., The Body Electric, Crosscurrents

Colloidal Silver — Its Uses Before 1938

The following is a list 37 of some of the (pre-1938) documented uses of silver, particularly in the colloidal form, for the treatment of various conditions and pathogens:

Anthrax Bacilli [2,3]	Axillae and Blind Boils of the Neck [10]
Appendicitis (post-op) [3]	B. Coli [2]

B. Coli Communis [7]
B. Dysenteria [2]
B. Pyocaneus [2]
B. Tuberculosis [7]
Bacillary Dysentery [4]
Bladder Irritation [12]
Blepharitis [13]
Boils [10]
Bromidrosis in Axille [12]
Bromidrosis in Feet [10]
Burns and Wounds of the Cornea [13]
Cerebro-spinal Meningitis [3,9]
Chronic Cystitis [10]
Chronic Eczema of Anterior Nares [10]
Chronic Eczema of Metus of Ear [10]
Colitis [4]
Cystitis [8]
Dacrocystitis [13]
Dermatitis suggestive of Toxaemia [4]
Diarrhoea [4]
Diptheria [3]
Dysentery [3,6]
Ear "Affections" [5]
Enlarged Prostrate [12]
Epiditymitis [10]
Erysipelas [3]
Eustachian Tubes (potency restored) [8]
Follicular Tonsilittis [10]
Furunculosis [3]
Gonococcus [7]
Gonorrhoea [10]
Gonorrhoeal Conjunctivitis [10]
Gonorrhoeal Opthalmia [13]
Gonorrhoeal Prostratic Gleet [11]
Haemorrhoids [12]
Hypopyon Ulcer [13]
Impetigo [10]
Infantile Disease [16]
Infected Ulcers of the Cornea [13]
Inflammatory Rheumatism [3]
Staphylococcus Pyogens Aureus [2]
Streptococci [7]
Subdues Inflammation [12]
Suppurative Appendicitis (post-op) [10]
Tinea Versicolor [10]
Tonsillitis [8]
Typhoid [3]
Typhoid Bacillus [14]

Influenza [11]
Interstitial Keratitis [13]
Intestinal troubles [6]
Lesion Healing [12]
Leucorrhoea [8]
Menier's Symptoms [8]
Nasal Catarrh [5]
Nasopharyngeal Catarrh (reduced) [8]
Oedematous enlargement of Turbinates
      without True Hyperplasia [9]
Offensive Discharge of Chronic
      Supporation in Otitis Media [10]
Ophthalmology [12]
Ophthalmic practices [5]
Para-Typhoid [3]
Paramecium [1]
Perineal Eczema [12]
Phlegmons [3]
Phlyctenular Conjunctivitis [10]
Pneumococci [2]
Pruritis Ani [12]
Puerperal Septicaemia [15]
Purulent Opthalmia of Infants [13]
Pustular Eczema of Scalp [10]
Pyorrhoea Alveolaris (Rigg's Disease) [8]
Quinsies [8]
Rhinitis [9]
Ringworm of the body [10]
Scarlatina [3]
Sepsis [16]
Septic Tonsillitis [10]
Septic Ulcers of the legs [10]
Septicaemia [5,8]
Shingles [8]
Soft Sores [10]
Spring Catarrh [10]
Sprue [6]
Staphyloclysin (inhibits) [2]
Staphylococcus Pyogenea [7]
Staphylococcus Pyogens Albus [2]
Ulcerative Urticaria [4]
Urticaria suggestive of Toxaemia [12]
Valsava's Inflammation [8]
Vincent's Angina [10]
Vorticella [1]
Warts [12]
Whooping Cough [8]

More recent articles have described silver being used to treat:

Adenovirus [5,23]

Asper Gillus Niger [18]

Bacillius Typhosus [21]

Bovine Rotavirus [23]

Candida Albicans [18]

Endamoeba Histolytica (Cysts) [24]

Escherichia Coli [17,18,21]

Legionella Pneumophila [17]

Poliovirus 1 (Sabin Strain) [23]

Pseudomonas Aeruginosa [17,18]

Salmonella [22]

Spore-Forming Bacteria [24]

Staphylococcus Aureus [17]

Streptococcus Faecalis [17]

Vegetative B. Cereus Cells [24]

The following is a documented list of silver resistant bacteria:

Citrobacter Freundii [20]

Enterobacter Cloacae [20]

Enterobacteriaceae (some strains) [19]

Escherichia Coli (some strains) [19]

Klebsiella Pneumoniae [20]

P. Stutzeri (some strains) [19]

Proteus Mirabilis [20]

Vegetative B. Cereus Spores [24]

Bibliographic References

[1] Bechhold, H. *Colloids in biology and medicine*, translated by J.G.M. Bullow., D. Van Nostrand Company; New York,1919, p.367.

[2] Ibid., p. 368.

[3] Ibid., p. 376.

[4] Searle, A.B. *The use of colloids in health and disease*. (Quoting from the British Medical Journal, May 12, 1917) E.P. Dutton & Company; New York 1919, p.82.

[5] Ibid., (Quoting from the British Medical Journal, Jan.15, 1917) p.83.

[6] Ibid., (Quoting Sir James Cantlie in the British Medical Journal, Nov.15, 1913)p. 83.

[7] Ibid., (Quoting Henry Crookes) p.70.

[8] Ibid., (Quoting J. Mark Hovell in the British Medical Journal, Dec.15, 1917) p.86.

[9] Ibid., (Quoting B. Seymour Jones) p. 86.

[10] Ibid., (Quoting C.E.A. MacLeod in Lancet, Feb.3, 1912) p. 83.

[11] Ibid., (Quoting J. MacMunn in the British Medical Journal, 1917,I, 685)p. 86.

[12] Ibid., (Quoting Sir Malcolm Morris in the British Medical Journal, May 12, 1917) p.85.

[13] Ibid., (Quoting A. Legge Roe in the British Medical Journal, Jan.16, 1915) p.83.

[14] Ibid., (Quoting W.J.Simpson in Lancet, Dec.12, 1914) pp.71-72.

[15] Ibid., (Quoting T.H.Anderson Wells in Lancet, Feb.16, 1918) p. 85.

[16] *Index-catalogue of the Library of the Surgeon General's Office United States Army*. United States Government Printing Office; Washington, v.IX, 1913, p. 628

17. Moyasar, T.Y.;Landeen, L.K.; Messina, M.C.; Kurtz, S.M.; Schulze, R.; and Gerba, C.P. *Disinfection of bacteria in water systems by using electrolytically generated copper, silver and reduced levels of free chlorine*. Found in Canadian Journal of Microbiology. The National Research Council of Canada' Ottawa, Ont., Canada, 1919, pp. 109-116.

18. Simonetti, N.; Simonetti, G.; Bougnol, F.; and Scalzo, M. *Electrochemical Ag+ for preservative use*. Article found in Applied and Environmental Microbiology. American Society for Microbiology; Washington, v.58,12,1992, pp.3834-3836.

19. Slawson, R.M.; Van Dyke, M.I.; Lee, H.; and Trevors, J.T. *Germanium and silver resistance, accumulation, and toxicity in microorganisms*. Article found in Plasmid. Academic Press, Inc.; San Diego, v.27, 1, 1992, 73-79.

20. Thurman, R.B. and Gerba, C.P. *The molecular mechanisms of copper and silver ion disinfection of bacteria and viruses*. A paper presented in the First International Conference on Gold and Silver in Medicine. The Silver Institute; Washington, v.18,4,1989, p. 295.

21. Ibid., p.299.

22. Ibid., p.300.

23. Ibid., p.301.

24. Ibid., p.302.

Appendix E

DHEA – The Mother of All Hormones

Alzheimer's, cancer, obesity, heart disease

What single weakness would you guess that aging, Alzheimer's disease, cancer, diabetes, heart disease, obesity, and senility have in common? According to Dr. Julian Whitaker's "Health and Healing Newsletter" (February 1994), it appears that low blood levels of DHEA (dihydroepiandrosterone) is the common factor!

What is DHEA?

DHEA is produced by our own adrenal glands, and is the most dominant steroid hormone in our body. Dr. William Regeison, the most noted of DHEA researchers, calls it "the mother hormone" because our body converts it upon demand into whatever hormone it needs, such as estrogen, testosterone, progesterone, corticosterone, etc. Blood levels of DHEA peak around age twenty. DHEA is the only hormone that declines in a linear fashion in both sexes, making it one of the most reliable markers of aging. By age eighty, blood levels are only 5 percent of what they were at age twenty. The decline of DHEA signals age-related diseases.

Preventing Breast Cancer

In a study on 5,000 apparently healthy women, it was discovered that 100 percent of the women developed and died of breast cancer that had blood levels of DHEA of less than 10 percent of that expected for their age group, and had sub-normal DHEA levels up to nine years before their cancer was diagnosed. All of the women with higher than average levels of DHEA remained cancer free. Other researchers picked up on this observation, and gave DHEA to rats who were inbred to develop breast cancer. DHEA blocked it! Arthur Schwartz, a researcher at Temple University in Philadelphia, found that DHEA blocks an enzyme called G6PD which promotes cancer cell division, as well as fat production.

Preventing heart disease and early death

Elizabeth Barrett-Connor, M.D., from the Department of Community and Family Medicine at the University of California School of Medicine in San Diego, tracked DHEA levels in 242 men aged twenty to seventy-nine for twelve years. She found that a 48 percent reduction in cardiovascular disease and a 36 percent reduction in mortality from any cause was correlated to a one hundred microgram per deciliter increase in DHEA sulfate blood levels. In the New England Journal of Medicine, she and other researchers concluded that even with people without heart disease, DHEA seems to protect against early death.

A 1988 study was done at John Hopkins in which rabbits with severe atherosclerosis were treated with DHEA. They had an almost 50 percent reduction in plaque size.

Lean-muscle Builder, Anti-obesity agent and Fat-burner

Arthur Schwartz, a researcher at Temple University in Philadelphia, found that DHEA blocks an enzyme called G6PD which promotes cancer cell division, as well as fat production. "There isn't any question," Schwartz says, "DHEA is a very effective anti-obesity agent."

According to Norman Applezweig of Progenics, Inc., DHEA gives an almost a fifty percent reduction in excess fat in mice. In fact, DHEA appears to be the first substance that, when laboratory tested, caused the loss of fat (as opposed to mere weight loss due to the breakdown of primary lean muscle tissue or fluid loss) without changing eating habits. Calories consumed were simply converted to heat rather than stored as fat. At the same time, it helped the body to produce lean muscle tissue.

For a month, doctors at the Medical College of Virginia gave daily doses of DHEA to five healthy men in their early twenties (none of the patients were obese, though four had excess body fat). Another five received a placebo. Diet and lifestyle remained the same. Result: In the DHEA group, the men's weight didn't change but body fat decreased 31 percent on average for four of the five (the one who didn't lose fat was already very lean). In the placebo group, there was no change. Best of all, fat seemed to have given way to muscle, the researchers report. And more: Blood levels of plaque-causing LDL cholesterol dropped about 7 percent.

A Memory Enhancer

In "Dr. Robert Atkins' Health Revelations" (January 1994), he states that DHEA has been shown to improve memory in aging mice, and there has been very active ongoing research on using DHEA against Alzheimer's. One study showed levels of DHEA in a group of Alzheimer's patients to be 48 percent lower than the control group.

Dr. Kenneth Bonnet, a research scientist in the Department of psychiatry at New York University School of Medicine, describes detailed testing with a forty-seven-year-old woman with lifelong multiple learning disabilities, low levels of memory retention, an inability to learn even the most simple information, and recurring headaches. Within one week of low doses of DHEA, the patient was retested and showed an improvement in recall ability and was sleeping more soundly. The woman also reported feeling an increase in clear thinking and ability to remember.

After one month, a higher dose of DHEA was given to the woman. Testing showed more advance ability to recall, with long-term memory increasing also. By the end of the testing period, she showed a marked increase in abilities. She was able to understand more clearly material presented to her and could apply that material, and could make judgments based on material presented to her. In addition, for the first time in her forty-seven years of life, was able to begin and continue a small business.

Reduce Prostate Problems

The prostate gland, like the ovaries, uterus, breasts, and testicles, is a hormone-sensitive gland. At age twenty, the prostate is about the size of a chestnut, but at age forty it undergoes a hormone-mediated growth spurt, causing difficult urination, weak flow and nighttime urination. At this time, testosterone levels have been declining. This is associated with an increase in the prostate of one of its metabolites, dihydro-testosterone. Of course, DHEA will help keep testosterone levels higher in the body.

Roughly 400,000 prostate surgeries occur annually. The death rate is 1 in 56 procedures. Eight percent are hospitalized within three months because of complications, 1 in 20 become impotent, and one in 5 will need another resection. Wow! I think I'll skip the operation and take a DHEA precursor in capsule form.

Several herbs can also remedy prostate problems (see Chapter Eight for more detail).

Why isn't DHEA treatment more popular?

Unfortunately, until January 1994, DHEA was available only in a synthetic form and only through doctors who would prescribe it. The problem until now has been that oral intake of any naturally occurring DHEA was somewhat ineffective due to breakdown in the digestive tract. This challenge has been overcome with the development of Proteusterone, a patented all-natural formula that combines specific precursors (those used in the production of DHEA) with a proprietary delivery system that allows for proper absorption and utilization.

Our introduction to DHEA

Patti first read about DHEA in a booklet entitled *Fat Burners*. It sounded too good to be true. In Patti's opinion, it was the best product mentioned in the book. However, the book went on to say that it was almost impossible to obtain, as it was developed synthetically and required a doctor's prescription. Then I read about it in Dr. Julian Whitaker's newsletter and he, too, raved about it but, also, said it was very difficult to obtain. Well, you can imagine our excitement when we were told that a new process had been developed by a company in Texas and that everyone could purchase a product which would stimulate the body's own production of DHEA. This capsule is a precursor contain-ing Dioscorea. When this precursor is taken with a meal, it mixes in your stomach with the fat and cholesterol in the meal and produces Pregnenolone, which can break down to DHEA or Progesterone, and these two hormones are used to produce any hormone your body needs. A diagram showing this progression is provided at the end of this appendix.

What also excited us was the unbelievable about of research that has been done on DHEA. Any doctor, or you, yourself, can go to "Dialgo Med11" (a computerized on-line search service) and have it do a search on "DHEA" and get an index of 40,186 articles. Hospitals should have access to this as well as any medical university. We have access to it through the University of Buffalo. Unbelievably, all but four articles are positive! We immediately started taking the product.

Will your body's natural production of DHEA shut down?

Anabolic, androgenic (male), estrogenic (female), and progestoid (gestational) steroid hormones do cause negative feedback inhibition. Steroid precursors like cholesterol, pregnenolone, and DHEA, which do not have much steroid activity, do not. The pituitary gland produces releasing hormones (peptides) which stimulate the testes, ovaries, and adrenal glands to produce steroid hormones. These steroid hormones circulate through the bloodstream to the hypothalamus in the brain which then sends a feedback signal to the pituitary, saying, "Make more" or "Make less." So feedback inhibition by steroids is controlled by the hypothalmic sensitivity to the steroid in question. Fortunately, the hypothalamus is quite specific. It does not recognize cholesterol, Pregnenolone, or DHEA as steroids and so does not down-regulate the pituitary's releasing hormones when these steroid precursors increase. Therefore, DHEA and Pregnenolone have few, if any, adverse side effects.

Some of DHEA's uses

- Increasing the blood level of DHEA decreases the stickiness of platelets, small particles in the blood that often clump together and cause heart attacks and strokes.
- It lowers blood pressure in animals.
- It has been shown to be helpful in cancer, Alzheimer's disease, multiple sclerosis, memory loss, chronic fatigue syndrome, and Parkinson's disease.
- It has been shown to increase the level of estrogen in women and testosterone in men to levels found in younger men and women. As such it just might be safer to supplement with DHEA in older men and women than with estrogen and testosterone. Women

have testified that increasing DHEA levels has reduced problems connected with their monthly cycles. Also, decrease in testosterone is related to prostate enlargement.

- DHEA lowers the blood cholesterol level, and studies are under way comparing DHEA to Mevacor, a cholesterol-lowering drug.

DHEA's effectiveness at ameliorating so many age-related diseases is consistent with its anti-aging properties. Think back to when you were twenty years old and had your highest blood levels of DHEA. What were your health problems then?

One Woman's Testimony of Relief

One friend of mine, found tremendous relief from problems produced within her body by her monthly menstrual cycle. Over the years she had been taken to the hospital three times with unbelievable cramps and pains so intense that she could not even move. After being on this precursor for a little over a month, all bodily warnings that her cycle was even beginning were gone and her mood and demeanor was 100% improved. She was ecstatic!

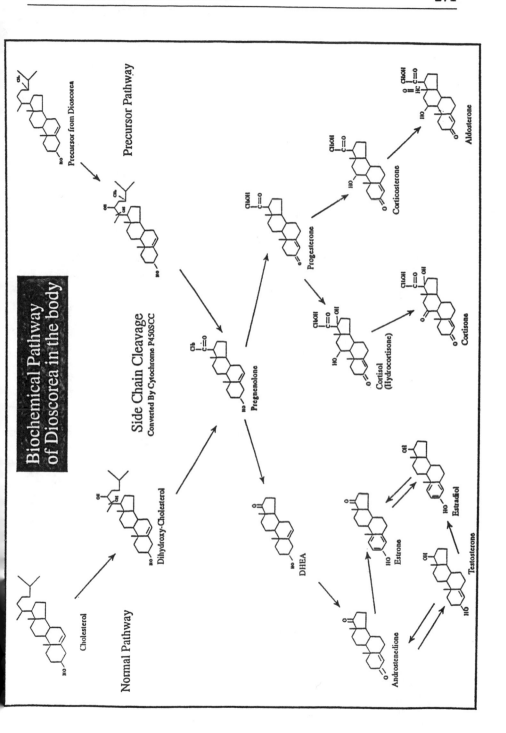

Biochemical Pathway of Dioscorea in the body

Renaissance Team Member

I wish to be listed as a member of the Renaissance Team. I agree to take responsibility to extend the Kingdom of God through the area(s) God has called me to work and serve. I will search the Bible for any principles which apply to that area. I will seek revelation from the Holy Spirit as to how to apply them. I will apply them under the anointing of the Holy Spirit. I will continue to be a learner. I will be willing to constantly set aside my preconceived ideas in order to be open to new things the Lord may be doing in His Church. I will move in faith in the power of God to accomplish His purpose through His Church of discipling the nations. I will not seek to dominate others but to serve them with the gifts which God has given to me.

_____ Please send me a certificate as a Renaissance Team Member and put me on a list to receive any mailings which may go out to this group.

Name _____

Address _____

City_____State _____ Zip _____

Phone: Home _____ Work _____ Fax_____

Mail to Covenant Enterprises (this is Mark & Patti's "for profit" company), 1431 Bullis Rd. Elma, N.Y. 14059 or fax to 716-652- 6961.

Quality of Life Questionnaire

Permission is given to copy this form to complete yourself and give a copy to a close friend to complete about you, also. Then average the scores together. It is good to do this every three to six months to see how you are improving.

1 - essentially none   2 - very little

3 - a fair amount   4 - a pretty good amount

5 - the full recommended amount

Area	Date	Date	Date	Date
Exercise				
Stretching				
Aerobic				
Strength-building				
Nourishment				
Eat the Genesis Diet				
Eat organic (or a superfood)				
Take vitamins regularly				
Take antioxidants				
Take herbs, as necessary				
Take enzymes or eat much raw foods				
Drink 6 - 8 glasses of pure water				
Take an immune system enhancer (e.g., aloe vera)				
Enhance DHEA levels				
Cleansing				
Fast regularly				
Maintain colon health				
Take acidophilus (or eat no meats, no antibiotics, or chlorine)				
Breathe fresh air				
Non-toxic environment				
Build immune system with aloe				

Area	Date	Date	Date	Date
Attitudes				
Live in faith, hope and love				
Live in joy and peace				
Laugh and enjoy life				
Recreation & quality bonding time				
Process emotions effectively				
Communicate openly and completely				
Pray for healing and health				
Take responsibility for own health				
Total score (of 27 items above)				

Maximum score is 135. Aim for at least 115.
A score above 81 indicates regeneration is taking place.
A score below 81 indicates degeneration is taking place.

The Thirty-Day Challenge

I challenge you to an experiment. For thirty days, practice the following healthy disciplines and see how you feel. I believe you will feel so much better that you will not go back to your old way of living. You may participate in Plan A only, or you may add Plan B and/or C.

Plan A: Basic 30-day challenge for everyone

1. Eat a minimum of 80% of your diet from the Genesis diet.
2. Exercise at least 20 minutes per day four days a week.
3. Drink six to eight glasses of pure water each day.
4. Forgive everyone for everything, and pray God's blessing upon them. Pray for healing, using the laying on of hands.
5. Take enzymes with each cooked meal to aid in digestion.
6. Take acidophilus first thing upon awakening to restore the proper flora to your intestines.
7. If you need to "kick start" your system because you have very low energy and intense food cravings, take some chromium and herbs.

Plan B: Additional Supplements

8. Take an all-natural multiple vitamin and a calcium supplement bonded to something your cells can easily assimilate.
9. Take an all-natural antioxidant.
10. Consume some excellent algae or other superfood daily.
11. Take a precursor to increase levels of DHEA in your bloodstream.
12. Take the 14-day colon cleanse program of herbs, which contains a four-day fast in the middle of it.
13. If you sense your immune system is weak, take a good quality aloe vera juice or capsule every day.

Plan C: Pure Air and Pure Water

For those seeking pure air and water, make sure a high quality air and water purifier are installed in your home.

To order a month's supply of any of the products mentioned above, contact the person who gave you this book or whose name is stamped on the order form at the back, or contact Mark and Patti Virkler (Covenant Enterprises) at 1-800-422-4816.

I Took the 30-Day Challenge!

Name _____ Phone _____

Address _____

City_____ State _____ Zip _____

I grant you permission to use my testimony if you desire. __ Yes __ No

Please change my name. ___ Yes ___ No

The dates of my 30-day challenge were from _____ through _____.

I was on ___ Plan A, ___ Plan B, ____ Plan C, with the following additions or deletions: _____

_____

_____

My Testimony _____

_____

_____

_____

_____

_____

_____

_____

_____

_____

_____

_____

_____

_____

_____

_____

_____

**Copy form and return to Communion With God Ministries,
1431 Bullis Rd., Elma, NY 14059**

Communion With God Ministries Order Form

1431 Bullis Road, Elma, N.Y. 14059
Order line only 1-800-466-6961 Other services 716-652-6990
Fax 716-652-6961

Visa Card - Master Card - American Express

Name _____ Phone _____

Address _____

City_____ State _____ Zip _____

All prices subject to change without notice.

Life Pack Order Form!

In taking responsibility for your own health, there is some basic life-changing knowledge which you just need to know and apply. That information can be found in the "Life Pack" listed below.

The key foundational books which everyone should own are:

#	BOOK	PRICE
	The McDougall Plan by John McDougall	$10.95
	McDougall's Medicine: A Challenging Second Opinion by John McDougall	$11.95
	The McDougall Health Supporting Cookbooks Vol. 1 & 2 by Mary McDougall	$9.95 each
	The Cancer Answer by A. E. Carter and Larry Lymphocyte	$10.95
	Counseled by God by Mark and Patti Virkler	$8.95
	Fast Your Way to Health by Lee Bueno	$8.99
	Power Healing by John Wimber	$14.95
	Your Personal Trainer by Ann Goodsell	$14.95
	Options: The Alternative Cancer Therapy Book by Richard Walters	$13.95
	Prescription for Nutritional Healing by James & Phyllis Balch	$16.95
	Disease Free by Matthew Hoffman, William LeGro and the editors of <u>Prevention Magazine</u>	$27.95

#	BOOK	PRICE
	Buy the complete **Life Pack** consisting of above 12 books valued at $160.44 for only $144.00, a 10% savings (all prices subject to change without notice). Applying the information in these books may take you a year, but could easily add ten years to your life, save you a $25,000 operation, and give you vibrant health throughout your life. So it is well worth your investment!	$144.00
	Eden's Health Plan - Go Natural! by Mark and Patti Virkler	$12.95
	Eden's Health Plan Teacher's Guide by Mark & Patti Virkler	$12.95
	Eden's Health Plan Video Cassettes by Mark Virkler (6 hrs)	$99.00
	Eden's Health Plan Audio Cassettes by Mark Virkler (6 hrs)	$19.95
	Communion With God Study Guide by Mark and Patti Virkler	$17.95
	Dialogue With God by Mark and Patti Virkler	$8.95
	Naturally Supernatural by Mark and Patti Virkler	$6.95
	The Flow of Life by Mark and Patti Virkler	$9.95
	Free listing of 50 other books written by Mark & Patti Virkler	Free
	Free information about Communion With God Ministries, a ministry headed by Mark Virkler	Free
	Information on an external degree from Christian Leadership University (Mark Virkler is the President of this University.)	Free
	The Anointing of the Holy Spirit by Peter Tan	$7.95
	The Cancer Battle Plan by Anne E. Frahm	$12.00
	Why Are You Poisoning Your Family by Kare Possick	$3.00
	The Antioxidants by Richard Passwater	$2.95
	Chromium Picolinate by Richard Passwater	$2.95
	Colloidal Silver by Canty and Baranowski CN	$3.50
	The New Superantioxidant - Plus by Richard Passwater	$2.95
More Helpful Tools The following items are in a "slide-rule" format which provides a lot of information in an easy-to-read style in a small space. Can be easily carried in your purse or briefcase for immediate reference wherever you are.		
	Eating Smart Guide – Features fast access to the facts on over 90 common foods and beverages. Shown for each item: calorie, sodium, fat, fiber, carbohydrate, and cholesterol counts. Back includes definitions of each nutrient, and recommended daily allowances for adults.	$2.00

#	BOOK	PRICE
	Less Fat Made Easy – Lists lower-fat alternatives for 75 everyday foods and drinks. Also includes quick instructions for finding fat contents in foods as well as a chart that lists recommended calorie and fat intake for various age groups.	$2.00
	Eating Out Nutrition Guide – Lets you quickly see the nutritional value - calorie, fat, protein, cholesterol, and sodium count - of over 100 popular restaurant choices. Includes: Coffee Shop/Diner; Oriental; Mexican; Italian; Steak and Seafood; Salad Bar; Delicatessen Items.	$2.00
	Low-Fat Food Finder – Pocket-size. The front has 4 steps to quickly find the dietary fat content of any packaged food. Simply check the food label, set the slide, and the fat rating appears in the window.	$1.50
	Lowering Your Cholesterol – Offers lower-cholesterol alternatives to 81 common high-cholesterol foods and beverages.	$2.00
	Facts on Fast Food – Nutritional lowdown on over 100 foods at today's most popular fast food restaurants. Quickly shows the calories, sodium, saturated fat, total fat, and cholesterol counts for main and side dishes from specific restaurants.	$2.00
	Recipe Substitutions: Your Guide to Healthier Cooking – Features over 60 great substitutes for common ingredients, as well as the benefit of each alternative choice.	$2.00
	Weight Management Food Diary – This 36-page guide helps you modify your behavior by using a food diary, understanding obstacles to weight loss, setting healthy eating goals, changing eating habits and maintaining healthy eating. Also pages for weight management records.	$3.00
	Step by Step: A Guide to Start You Walking – This 36-page guide lets you set your walking goals, then log 6 weeks of progress. It contains: daily checklists of goals reached; daily motivational tips; aerobic facts and monitoring techniques; strength training exercises; warm up and cool-down stretches; and much more.	$1.50
	70 Great Stress Busters – Offers 70 smart things to keep daily stress down. Peel-off adhesive-back strip lets you hand it up wherever you need it most: on the wall, file cabinet, bulletin board or refrigerator.	$1.00
	Stress Card – A wallet-size card. Place your thumb on a specific are for ten seconds, and the area turns various colors for stressed, tense, normal and calm.	$3.00
	Save! Buy one of each of the above items and receive the **entire package for $18.00** — a savings of $4.00!	$18.00
	TOTAL	

Resource Directory Order Form

Informational packs on the following resources may obtained from:
Covenant Enterprises, 1431 Bullis Rd. Elma, N.Y. 14059
(716) 629-8472.

Please send me the following informational packets:
($3.00 per pack)

____ Information on an outstanding multiple vitamin.

____ Information on non-toxic natural household cleansers and skin
care items.

____ Information on chromium and herbs supplements.

____ Information on herb combinations for specific problems.

____ Information on high-quality aloe to build the immune system,
pycnogenol, the super-antioxidant, and colloidal silver.

____ Information on a DHEA precursor.

____ Information on blue-green algae capsules, acidophilus and
enzymes.

____ Information on a good air filter.

____ Information on a good water filter.

____ Information on the Living Water System.

____ Information on how to make some extra money so I can afford all
these products.

Include $3.00 per informational pack ordered. I have included $_____
with this order.

Total enclosed _____

Please ship to:

Name _____ Phone _____

Address _____

City_____ State _____ Zip _____

See following page for ordering information.

Ordering Information

To order the informational packs from the previous page you may contact Covenant Enterprises, 1431 Bullis Rd. Elma, N.Y. 14059; or call us at (716) 629-8472.

If there is an address listed below you may contact it for more personalized assistance

Bibliography

Albrecht, William. *The ALBRECHT Papers Volume I*. Ed. Charles Walters, Jr. Kansas City, MO: Acres U.S.A., 1975.

Albrecht, William. *The ALBRECHT Papers Volume II*. Ed. Charles Walters, Jr. Kansas City, MO: Acres U.S.A., 1975.

Balch, James F. and Phyllis A. Balch. *Prescription for Nutritional Healing*. Garden City Park, NY: Avery Publishing Group, 1990.

Batmanghelidj, F. *Your Body's Many Cries for Water*. Falls Church, VA: Global Health Solutions, 1992.

Bland, Jeffrey. *Digestive Enzymes*. New Canaan, CT: Keats Publishing, 1983.

"Blood and Lymph." *The World Book Encyclopedia of Science*. 1989 ed.

Brennan, Barbara Ann. *Hands of Light*. New York: Bantam, 1987.

Bricklin, Mark and Maggie Spilner, eds. *Walking for Health*. Emmaus, PA: Rodale Press, 1992.

Bueno, Lee. *Fast Your Way to Health*. Springdale, PA: Whitaker House, 1991.

Buhler, Rich. *Pain and Pretending*. Nashville, TN: Thomas Nelson, 1991.

Cameron, Ewan and Linus Pauling. *Cancer and Vitamin C*. Philadelphia, PA: Camino Books, 1993.

Carper, Jean. *The Food Pharmacy*. New York: Bantam Books, 1988.

Carter, Albert Earl & Larry Lymphocyte. *The Cancer Answer*. Fountain Hills, AZ: A.L.M. Publishers, 1988.

Cassano, Kimberly Bright. *Candida Elimination Program*. Clearwater, FL: Kimberly Bright Cassano Enterprises, 1993, 1994.

Castleman, Michael. *The Healing Herbs*. Emmaus, PA: Rodale Press, 1991.

Diamond, Harvey and Marilyn. *Fit for Life*. New York: Warner Books, 1985.

Dollinger, Malin, Ernest H. Rosenbaum, and Greg Cable. *Everyone's Guide to Cancer Therapy*. Kansas City, MO: Andrews and McMeel, 1991.

"Don't Let Soil Compaction Squeeze Your Profits". Indianapolis, IN: Elanco Products.

Dossey, Larry. *Healing Words*. New York: HarperCollins Publishers, 1993.

Frahm, Anne E. with David J. Frahm. *A Cancer Battle Plan*. Colorado Springs, CO: Pinon Press, 1992.

Frank, Jerome D. *Persuasion and Healing*. New York: Schocken, 1961.

Gardner, Joseph, ed. *Eat Better, Live Better*. Pleasantville, NY: The Reader's Digest Association, Inc., 1982.

Gerson, Max. *A Cancer Therapy*. Bonita, CA: THe Gerson Institute, 1990.

Glassburn, Vicki. *Who Killed Candida?* Brushton, NY: TEACH Service, 1991.

Goodrich, Janet. *Natural Vision Improvement*. Berkeley, CA: Celestial Arts, 1986.

Goodsell, Ann. *Your Personal Trainer*. Des Moines, IA: Better Homes and Gardens Books, 1994.

Graham, Keith, et al. *Biology: God's Living Creation*. Pensacola, FL: A Beka Books, 1986.

Grover, Linda. *August Celebration*. Carson City, NV: Gilbert, Hoover & Clarke, 1993.

Hart, Archibald D. *Adrenalin & Stress*. Waco, TX: Word, 1986.

Hayes, Norvel. *How to Live and Not Die*. Tulsa, OK: Harrison House, 1986.

Hickey, Marilyn. *Your Total Health Handbook*. Denver, CO: Marilyn Hickey Ministries, 1993.

Hoffman, Matthew, William LeGro. *Disease Free*. Emmaus, PA: Rodale Press, 1993.

Hunter, Charles and Frances. *Handbook for Healing*. Kingwood, TX: Hunter Ministries, 1987.

Igram, Cass. *Killed on Contact*. Cedar Rapids, IA: Literary Visions Publishing, 1992.

Jensen, Bernard. *Arthritis, Rheumatism and Osteoporosis*. Escondido, CA: Bernard Jensen Enterprises, 1986.

Jensen, Bernard. *Breathe Again Naturally*. Escondido, CA: Bernard Jensen Enterprises, 1983.

Jensen, Bernard. *Doctor-Patient Handbook*. Escondido, CA: Bernard Jensen Enterprises, 1976.

Jensen, Bernard. *Iridology Simplified*. Escondido, CA: Bernard Jensen Enterprises, 1980.

Jensen, Bernard. *Love, Sex & Nutrition*. Garden City Park, NY: Avery Publishing Group, 1988.

Jensen, Bernard. *Tissue Cleansing Through Bowel Management*. Escondido, CA: Bernard Jensen Enterprises, 1981.

Jensen, Bernard. *World Keys to Health and Long Life*. Escondido, CA: Bernard Jensen Enterprises, 1975.

Josephson, Elmer A. *God's Key to Health and Happiness*. Old Tappan, NJ: Fleming H. Revell, 1976.

Keith, Velma J. and Monteen Gordon. *The How to Herb Book*. Pleasant Grove, UT: Mayfield Publications, 1984.

Lin, David J. *Free Radicals and Disease Prevention*. New Canaan, CT: Keats Publishing, 1993.

Lindsay, Gordon. *The Reason Why Christians Are Sick and How They May Get Well*. Dallas, TX: Christ for the Nations.

Lynes, Barry. *The Healing of Cancer*. Queensville, Ontario: Marcus Books, 1989.

Manning, Kenneth R. "Pasteur, Louis." *World Book Encyclopedia*. 1989 ed.

McDougall, John A. *McDougall's Medicine: A Challenging Second Opinion*. Clinton, NJ: New Win Publishing, 1985.

McDougall, John A. *The McDougall Plan*. Clinton, NJ: New Win Publishing, 1983.

McDougall, John A. *The McDougall Program*. New York: Penguin Books,

McMillen, S. I. *None of These Diseases*. Westwood, NJ: Fleming H. Revell, 1963.

Mullins, Eustace. *Murder by Injection*. Staunton, VA: The National Council for Medical Research, 1988.

Omartian, Stormie. *Greater Health God's Way*. Waco, TX: Word, 1984.

Osteen, Dodie. *Healed of Cancer*. Houston, TX: John Osteen, 1986.

Padus, Emrika. *The Complete Guide to Your Emotions & Your Health*. Emmaus, PA: Rodale Press, 1986.

Passwater, Richard A. *Chromium Picolinate*. New Canaan, CT: Keats Publishing, 1992.

Passwater, Richard A. *Chromium Picolinate*. New Canaan, CT: Keats Publishing, 1992.

Passwater, Richard A. *The New Superantioxidant - Plus*. New Canaan, CT: Keats Publishing, 1992.

Possick, Kare. *Why Are You Poisoning Your Family?* Madeira Beach, FL: Kare Possick, 1994.

Reams, Carey A. with Cliff Dudley. *Choose Life or Death*. Tampa, FL: Holistic Laboratories, 1990.

Ritter, Lee. *Aloe Vera: A Mission Discovered*. Northglenn, CO: Lee Ritter, 1993.

Scarborough, Peggy. *Healing Through Spiritual Warfare*. Shippensburg, PA: Treasure House, 1994

Shelton, Herbert M. *Fasting Can Save Your Life*. Tampa, FL: American Natural Hygiene Society, 1978.

Siegel, Bernie S. *Love, Medicine & Miracles*. New York: Harper and Row, 1986.

Swope, Mary Ruth. *Gree Leaves of Barley*. Melbourne, FL: National Preventive Health Services, 1987.

Tenney, Louise. *Today's Herbal Health*. Provo, UT: Woodland Health Books, 1983.

Tessler, Gordon S. *Clean and Unclean Foods*. Raleigh, NC: Trumpets of Zion Ministries, 1991.

Tessler, Gordon S. *Did God Change His Mind?* Raleigh, NC: Trumpets of Zion Ministries, 1991.

Virkler, Henry A. *Speaking Your Mind Without Stepping on Toes*. Scripture Press Publications, 1991.

Vogel, H. C. A. *The Nature Doctor*. New York: Instant Improvement, 1952, 1991.

Walker, N. W. *Become Younger*. Prescott, AZ: Norwalk Press, 1949.

Walker, N. W. *The Natural Way to Vibrant Health*. Prescott, AZ: Norwalk Press, 1972.

Walker, Norman W. *Natural Weight Control*. Prescott, AZ: Norwalk Press, 1981.

Wallis, Arthur. *God's Chosen Fast*. Fort Washington, PA: Christian Literature Crusade, 1968.

Walters, Charles Jr. and C. J. Fenzau. *An Acres U.S.A. Primer*. Raytown, MO: Acres U.S.A., 1979.

Walters, Richard. *Options: The Alternative Cancer Therapy*. Garden City Park, NY: Avery Publishing Group, 1993.

Weinberger, Stanley. *Parasites: An Epidemic in Disguise*. Larkspur, CA: Healing Within Products, 1993.

Wheeler, Philip A. and Ronald B. Ward. *Non-Toxic Farming: A Handbook*. TransNational AGronomy, 1989.

Williams, Redford and Virginia Williams. *Anger Kills*. New York: Random House, 1993.

Willix, Robert D. *Maximum Health*. Baltimore, MD: Agora, 1993.

Wimber, John, with Kevin Springer. *Power Healing*. New York: Harper and Row, 1987.

Zehr, Albert. *Healthy Steps*. Burnaby, Canada: Abundant Health Publishers, 1990